Gordon's Guide to the Surgical Morbidity and Mortality Conference

Gordon's Guide to the Surgical Morbidity and Mortality Conference

Leo A. Gordon, MD, FACS
General Surgeon
Los Angeles, California

HANLEY & BELFUS, INC./ Philadelphia
MOSBY/ St. Louis • Baltimore • Boston • Chicago • London
Philadelphia • Sydney • Toronto

Publisher: HANLEY & BELFUS, INC.
Medical Publishers
210 S. 13th Street
Philadelphia, PA 19107
(215) 546-7293

North American and worldwide sales and distribution:

MOSBY
11830 Westline Industrial Drive
St. Louis, MO 63146

In Canada: Times Mirror Professional Publishing, Ltd.
130 Flaska Drive
Markham, Ontario L6G 1B8
Canada

GORDON'S GUIDE TO THE SURGICAL
MORBIDITY AND MORTALITY CONFERENCE   ISBN 1-56053-103-7

1994 by Hanley & Belfus, Inc. All rights reserved. No part of this book may be reproduced, reused, republished, or transmitted in any form or by any means without written permission of the publisher.

Library of Congress catalog card number   93-79226

Last digit is the print number: 9 8 7 6 5 4 3 2 1

THIS GUIDE IS DEDICATED TO RICHARD YEE.

Contents

Preface vii
Acknowledgments xi

1. The Philosophy of the M and M Conference 1
2. Surgical Complications 3
3. The Format of the M and M Conference 7
   The Moderator 9
   The Room 11
   The Audience 13
4. The Case Presentation 21
   Preparation 21
   Data Retrieval 22
   Classification of Complications 27
   Presentation Mechanics: Text, Film, and Slides 30
   Questions, Answers, and Discussion 33
   The Case in Context 36
   The Summary 37
   The Attending Summary 37
   Damage Control 38
   Special Circumstances 41
5. The Presentation of Laparoscopic Complications 45
6. The Unwritten Rules of M and M 51
7. Dress and Demeanor 53
8. The Surgical Notebook 55
9. Competition 59
10. Miscellanea Morbidita 61
    Trademarks 61
11. The Spirit of M and M: Surgery 101 67

Epilogue 69

Appendix 1:   Richard Yee   71

Appendix 2:   The M and M Checklist   75

Appendix 3:   How to Make M and M More Interesting:
              A 10-Point Plan   77

Appendix 4:   Great Moments in the History
              of the Surgical M and M Meeting   81

Appendix 5:   An Inquiry into the Origin of Surgical
              Academia   85

Preface

After skewering a poorly prepared resident with a vitriolic comment at our weekly morbidity and mortality meeting, I was chastised by the moderator with the following comment:

"Look, this is not a contest!!"

I have a great deal of respect for the surgical professoriate. I respect any cadre of American medicine that can state: ". . . laparoscopic cholecystectomy in humans should be confined to specialized centers that participate in current or planned prospective studies designed to optimize the technique and carefully refine its indications."* Nevertheless, I never let this respect cloud my judgment of their formal comments or actions, particularly in the presence of surgical residents.

The professor who made this comment was dead wrong. The weekly morbidity and mortality conference **is** a contest. It is a contest to see who can get the patient better, quicker with fewer mistakes. It is a contest whose winners demonstrate the best of surgical thought and action. Those winners use the morbidity and mortality conference to see who, in this contest, is playing by the rules. You may remember the concept of playing by rules. Although it fell out of fashion in the mid 1980s, it is making a comeback. The rules of the contest are the rules of clinical surgery.

This is a contest that I like to win. Winning is important. Winning is a basic part of surgery. Every morning we walk into a locker room, put on uniforms, and join a team. The tone is set for winning even before our "games" begin. It is that spirit of winning that has led me to write this book. During my early surgical education, I

---

*Cuschieri, Alfred, et al: Laparoscopic cholecystectomy. Am J Surg 159:273, 1990

had often wished that there were a book describing the rules and format of the weekly morbidity and mortality meeting. I was impressed that in all of the tomes of surgical knowledge, no such document was present. No professor, fellow, resident, or intern had ever sat down and spelled out the framework for this most important hour of the surgical week. As with some great tribal tradition, the rules and approaches were handed down orally from resident to resident.

In amongst my surgical papers is a worn and frayed edition of *The Elements of Style* by William Strunk, Jr. Strunk was a professor of English at Cornell in the 1920s. What he did was remarkable for its need and simplicity. He saw the need for a brief collection of the essential points of English grammar and composition. In an unusual move for a professor, he did not attempt to write the "definitive" textbook. He was too practical for that. He boiled everything down to essential guidelines of English in 43 pages! He had the book privately printed for his students.*

I am not the William Strunk, Junior of clinical surgery. I more closely resemble the Biff Loman of clinical surgery, but that's another story. I felt a similar need to boil down and to codify the guidelines for effective presentations at morbidity and mortality meetings just as Strunk had done for English usage.

This guide is the distilled and refined thought from hundreds of morbidity and mortality meetings across the country in a variety of surgical departments in which I have been privileged to participate as an intern, a resident, a fellow, and an attending surgeon. It takes impressions and guidelines from surgical education programs in the East, the West, the Midwest, and the South, and creates a disciplined approach to the meeting.

This document is a guide, not a rule book. For that reason it should not be confused with such surgical maxims as: "Never let the sun rise or set . . .", or "Always drain if . . ." It presents general guidelines to help the resident at any level to prepare for and present to the weekly morbidity and mortality meeting.

Although I am a professional general surgeon, I am an amateur surgical educator. There is something free and refreshing about be-

---

*White, E. B: The Elements of Style, 3rd ed. New York, Macmillan Publishing, 1979.

PREFACE

ing an amateur. The amateur spirit seems to have been beaten out of many of today's surgical educators. This spirit is a spirit of innovation, fun, and practical thought that has often led to great advances.

The true leader is an amateur in the proper, original sense of the word. The amateur (from Latin *amateur*, "lover"; from *amore*, "to love") does something for the love of it. He pursues his enterprise not for money, not to please the crowd, not for professional prestige or for assured promotion and retirement at the end—but because he loves it. If he can't help doing it, it's not because of the forces pushing from behind but because of his fresh, amateur's vision of what lies ahead.*

Gordon's Guide to the Surgical Morbidity and Mortality Conference does not represent the official policies of any Department of Surgery, or of the Office of Shapiro and Gordon (as a California Corporation). It does not reflect the managerial policies of Gordon's Army and Navy Store, their employees or their families. Those families and heirs are exempt from any implied contract, *force majeure, nolo contendere,* or other stuff.

Enjoy this guide. And remember, as Halsted said:

"We were dry when we closed . . . "

Leo A. Gordon, M.D., FACS
Los Angeles, California

---

*Boorstin, Daniel J: "The Amateur Spirit and Its Enemies." Hidden History. New York, Vintage Books, 1987.

Acknowledgments

This guide has many contributors. It is an assimilation and distillation of hundreds of morbidity and mortality meetings that I have attended since 1971 when I began my clinical rotations in medical school. I was and still am fascinated by this meeting, its actions, and the give-and-take that it generates. I took something away from each meeting, and stored those somethings until now. I categorized them and recorded them. Only lately have I had the time or the inclination to formalize them into this Guide.

I have felt a need to write such a guide because I have observed a gradual decline in the importance of the morbidity and mortality meeting within the surgical residency. It seems that the most important aspects of surgical life are most intensely and clearly stated in the forum of the morbidity and mortality meeting.

Woven into the fabric of the text are ideas and comments from the people with whom I have worked. And what an assortment those people represent! Professors, residents, medical students, nurses, fellows from all over the world—the spectrum of surgical activity in several large medical centers.

Singular contributions stand out. I have maintained close contact with three colleagues, all refugees from the 1960s who weathered the storm of Boston surgical training in the 1970s. This sisyphean task—a Boston surgical residency—was a crucible, the central event of which was the weekly morbidity and mortality meeting. These colleagues, in one way or another, helped me to understand the essence of the meeting. They helped me to refine my own skills and to use those skills within the meeting format. These colleagues were, and still are, invaluable to me in infusing a spirit of enthusiasm and fun into the ongoing assessment of surgery as an art and a science.

Dr. Allan Silberman, biochemist and surgical oncologist, was at my side during those testy morbidity and mortality meetings in Boston. I am indebted to him for his support during the writing of this Guide, and for his criticisms of the original text. He has tempered many of my points with the caution and restraint for which he is known. He is the only true professor of surgery I have ever met.

Who better than a Harvard-educated surgeon to give me insight into the mind and machinations of the surgical professoriate? Dr. Timothy Lepore, Harvard College 1962, Tufts Medical School 1968, currently Chief Surgeon, Nantucket Cottage Hospital, is a friend and surgical colleague in the truest sense. His oblique view of surgical life gave me the first inkling that the morbidity and mortality meeting could be valuable. Rather than using the meeting as a vehicle for professorial politics, Dr. Lepore created an educational model that found life at the weekly meeting. The child of a professor, encouraged to be a professor, brought up in a family of professors—who better to guide me into the depths of professorial inanity than one from their own ranks?

Dr. David Cossman's counsel and text corrections were particularly helpful in the section on understanding the nature of professional interplay at the morbidity and mortality meeting. His recollection of the Surgical Notebook and its value to the surgical resident helped to frame that section. It is of note that during his review of the manuscript, he never once brought up his Yale B.A. in literature (a document I personally have never seen). The spirit of this text is, to a large degree, the spirit of Dr. Cossman. That spirit of hard work and dispassionate assessment of that work is the essence of progress within the field of surgery.

I also owe a great debt to my partner and confidant, Professor Stephen J. Shapiro. A surgical partner is many things—mentor, colleague, advisor, and friend. I learned surgery during my residency. I became a surgeon under Dr. Shapiro's tutelage. Under his guidance, I built a modest practice. His unique views on the night-time treatment of gastrointestinal bleeding, bowel obstructions, and early appendicitis will be the subject of another text. (Unfortunately, the title "At Dawn We Slept" has already been used.) Dr. Shapiro is

ACKNOWLEDGMENTS

a busy surgeon whose income (distributed through a unique formula that allows me to become a full partner in 25 years) allowed me to purchase the computer on which this Guide was written.

The thoughts and comments of these colleagues became an intertwined whole that was a great stimulus to keep writing. All of these men have surgical spirit—a love and respect for surgery that transcends all specialties. They have carried that same spirit into their practices as attending surgeons. Their hospitals and patients are better off for it.

The real debt I owe, however, is to the legions of surgical residents who, week after week, around the world, prepare for and present surgical complications to their own meetings. My hope is that this Guide improves those presentations and in so doing improves surgical care.

Leo A. Gordon, M.D., FACS

Nihil est tam insigne, nec tam ad diurnit atem memoriae stabile, quam id, in quo aliquid offenderis.

Cicero De Oratore, I, 129

Nothing stands out so conspicuously, or remains so firmly fixed in our memory, as something in which we have blundered.

1

The Philosophy of the M and M Conference

Traumatologists speak of a "golden hour" after injury—an hour during which a surgeon has the opportunity, through skill and intelligence, to stave off the devastating effects of trauma. There is an analogy to that golden hour in surgical education—the morbidity and mortality meeting. Just as the trauma surgeon uses surgical skills to fight off injury, so must the resident use intellectual skills to fight off the injurious forces of surgical ignorance that lead to surgical complications. The morbidity and mortality meeting is the golden hour of surgical education.

The spirit of the morbidity and mortality meeting is the spirit of intellect, competition, showmanship, roundsmanship, and medical debate. It is the last bastion of this debate in medicine today. In this arena, the short can outwit the tall, the not-so-intelligent can outwit the intelligent, and, most important, the resident can outwit the attending. Surgical residents have the opportunity (and, many surgical educators feel, the responsibility) to rise above their station in life. During the meeting, they are on a plane with every surgeon in the room. The surgical resident is no longer the ill-prepared, sleep-deprived, half-starved, marginally motivated wretch who his colleagues think he is. He is the presenter at the morbidity and mortality meeting. He is center stage. As they say in Vegas, "He's playing the big room."

This hour is the most important hour of the surgical week.

During this hour residents have the opportunity to intellectually go one-on-one with the entire division. They have the chance to prove themselves in the sphere of clinical surgery. It is the only time when one can dispassionately and scientifically dissect an error and learn how to avoid that error in the future. It is an hour that, if it is to be beneficial to all who attend, must be highly regarded by every member of the surgical team.

The educational underpinning of the morbidity and mortality meeting is that after 5 years a resident will see common complications occur, and, **because of this conference,** will be able to anticipate and deal with them in a timely, responsible, surgically acceptable manner. It is further assumed that if an uncommon complication occurs, the resident will have achieved a level of surgical sophistication to know when and where to get help.

Just as there is an art and science to surgery, so is there an art and science to preparing, coordinating, and presenting at the morbidity and mortality meeting. The key to a successful meeting for all involved (presenter and audience) is an understanding of the elements of the conference and the interplay among those elements:

    Elements to be mastered are:
    1. What is a Complication?
    2. The Morbidity and Mortality Format
    3. The Case to be Presented
    4. The Audience

The resident who understands and masters these elements and who weaves them into a stimulating, insightful, and interesting presentation has mastered the art and science of the morbidity and mortality conference.

2

Surgical Complications

What is a surgical complication?

The usual course of events in surgery is that a patient presents with what is thought to be a surgical disease. That disease may be treated surgically. The patient then recovers and is dismissed from the hospital. If any problems arise during the 30 days following an operation, that event is considered to be a complication. Those events are usually recorded by the surgical team and presented to the morbidity and mortality meeting for discussion.

The term *complication* is quite specific. The Latin verb *plicare* was used to describe an intertwining of materials in weaving. Adding the prefix *com* meant that different materials were woven together, or more specifically, intertwined. The resulting fabrics were more difficult to make and were referred to as *complicatus*. The verb *complicare* was used to describe the action of weaving together an intricate fabric made up of differing elements. As with many other words in our language, this word was taken from a trade and came to be used to describe life events. Events that had several strains or themes that had many elements were labeled *complicated*. Difficult weaving situations were thus transposed to difficult life situations.

Surgical complications are events that arise during the 30 days following surgery that are difficult issues intertwined with the procedure that was performed. Any event that deviates from the anticipated uneventful recovery from surgery is, technically, a complication. This covers the entire spectrum from a red intravenous line site causing pain to an acute pulmonary embolus causing death. Everything in between is a complication.

How are complications reported?

If a complication occurs while the patient is in the hospital, it is noted and recorded. The chief resident or senior resident on that service usually does the recording. This list is then passed on to the surgical department where it is codified. Once recorded, complications are then selected for discussion. Which complications are selected depends on a number of factors.

If a complication occurs outside of the hospital and does not require readmission of the patient, it is generally lost. If the patient is readmitted for a surgical complication within the 30-day time limit, the complication is usually reported and presented for discussion.

Ideally, the complications selected should be chosen for their teaching value or for their unusual nature. All complications should be recorded, but all do not necessarily require discussion.

A recent meeting I attended devoted 25 minutes to discussion of a wound infection following a breast biopsy, while a re-bleed following gastrectomy, an enterocutaneous fistula following small bowel resection, and a trauma death were squeezed into the end of the hour. Although pertinent teaching points can be made from any complication, a sense of prioritization is needed to hold the interest of the audience.

It is a natural tendency of humans, particularly *homo surgiensis*, to want to "bury" some complications. Admitting and discussing one's errors in a peer-group setting are difficult for some surgeons. One common method of burying is not to report a frequent or expected complication. There is a lingering misconception among some surgeons that because a complication is anticipated, it is, therefore, not a complication. Such an approach is a naive attempt to deflect criticism. It is intellectually dishonest, and, frankly, foolish.

SURGICAL COMPLICATIONS

During the performance of cases, especially urgent ones, situations may arise that increase the incidence of certain complications. A pelvic abscess following a ruptured appendix, a postoperative bowel obstruction following extensive adhesiolysis, and a rebleed after a gastrectomy in a patient with thrombocytopenia are all anticipated complications. When they occur, although anticipated, **they are still complications and should be reported.** The fact that they are common or even anticipated does not alter the fact that they represent a deviation from normal recovery.

The skeins of medical politics and practice infiltrate most areas of a medical center. Rarely, though quite obviously, they can influence the morbidity and mortality list. Countless times have I seen my weary colleagues sit through presentations of their *errata*, while greater errors of others sit unlisted or unreported. The reasons for this are complex and outside the realm of this work.

Once a complication is recognized and reported, it must be classified. This process of classification is a basic part of preparing the case and is discussed in Chapter 4, "The Case Presentation."

Vigilance by the moderator of the meeting or by the chief of surgery sets the tone for a fair presentation and categorization of all surgical complications.

3

The Format of the M and M Conference

Research into the seminal documents of the surgical literature reveals the origin of the morbidity and mortality meeting. In the Edwin Smith Papyrus, the comment on Case XVI states:

" . . . if the set bone festers, and the slave suffers, the conclave of elders will convene and deliberate lest the healer know not of his error"*

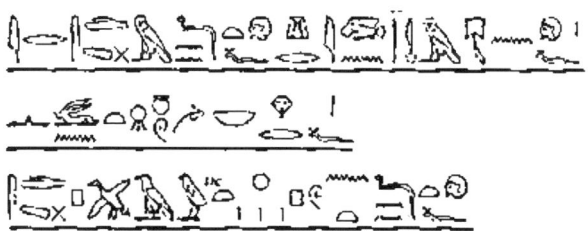

---

*Breasted, James Henry: The Edwin Smith Surgical Papyrus. Chicago, IL, The University of Chicago Press, 1930, p. 415. The commentary on Case XVI has been subject to multiple interpretations over the years. My interpretation of this commentary has wide support in the surgical-archaeological community.

Today's "conclave of elders" in most departments is a pastiche of surgeons with different levels of skill, dedication, training, and experience. There is also a great age differential. One might find such an audience difficult to present to. This *gemisch* of surgical backgrounds at every morbidity and mortality meeting is precisely why the meeting is so valuable. Multiple views of common surgical problems are a great educational tool, even if some of those views are wrong or outdated.

The resident must present to the middle ground. This accomplishes two things. It gives the informed surgeon a sense of superiority. It gives the uninformed surgeon a sense of education. The audience may range from superspecialized "lab rats" to senescent nursing home types whose last lucid thought occurred when Lindbergh landed. Accept this as a challenge of the presentation.

The format of the morbidity and mortality conference has evolved over the years. It has evolved into a format that is similar to that of a legal deposition.* There are rules. There are custom and habit. There may be levity, but there is also underlying intent and purpose. The intent is to educate. The purpose is to expose faulty or illogical reasoning and to prevent it in the future.

Understanding the format of the conference is essential to mastering the conference. This is true for the presenter as well as the audience. If the presenting resident does not understand the construct, the presentation will be choppy and aimless. If the audience does not understand it, the questions will be poorly framed and illogical.

Although this format is generally well accepted, there is variation around the country. The moderator of the conference has the obligation to follow the format. In smaller meetings with poor attendance, these become loose guidelines rather than rules of order. In larger meetings, a strict format is essential. Such a format fosters orderly thought on the part of the presenting resident. It also lets the audience know when it can speak and question. Finally, it allows the responsible surgeon to distill his thoughts as the discussion progresses.

In keeping with the general decline of manners in America, some members of the audience may not respect this format. When the debate over surgical principle and practice becomes heated, the presenter may be interrupted. Those attendings lacking restraint may make their comments too early. Those lacking knowledge may not

---

*Do not ask me how I know this.

Effective Format for the Surgical Morbidity and Mortality Conference

1. The complication is stated and classified.
2. The case is presented. This includes:
   a. A narrative of the case
   b. A review of studies pertinent to the case
   c. A review of the surgical procedure
   d. The chronology of the complication
   e. The treatment of the complication
3. Questions about the case and the complication are taken from the audience.
4. The case is discussed by the presenter **in the context of the surgical literature**
5. The responsible attending surgeon comments on the case.

comment at all. The moderator is the "keeper of the format." He must control the conference, lest it degenerate into a pitched battle.

Who is the moderator?

THE MODERATOR

At the **precise hour** of the conference, the surgeon in charge welcomes the audience. Who is this surgeon who runs the conference? It varies in different parts of the country. In the East, the chief resident runs the conference. This is the format I support. The chief resident year is a year unlike any other in a surgeon's life. It is the culmination of formal surgical education. Running such a conference contributes to his knowledge, develops organizational skills, and improves his ability to speak clearly in a group setting. Because he has major operative responsibilities, the presentation of the complications probably means more to him than to anyone else assembled.

If chief residents are to confront the daily problems of clinical surgery, this conference is an ideal training ground. The need to field unexpected questions and to master details of many cases, and the opportunity to actually feel responsible and involved in the problems of a busy surgical service contribute to surgical maturity. If a chief resident runs a morbidity and mortality conference for a year, his oral boards will assume the stress level of a goodnight kiss.

In many areas of the country, the chief of surgery runs the conference. Many people support this arrangement, as do many members of the Association for Surgical Education.* This setup keeps the chief of surgery in touch with his department, an increasingly difficult task. We no longer have chiefs of surgery in the classic sense. We now have departmental CEO's, and they have about as much of a chance at recognizing an intern as they do of winning a lottery. One way of keeping a chief a real chief in the classic educational sense is to make him clinically aware of his department. What greater way can there be than to run a weekly meeting, the heart and soul of which are daily surgical and clinical decision making?

Running the morbidity and mortality conference keeps up the clinical skills of the chief of surgery. He becomes a visible entity, not a corporate phantom. Such an arrangement has a good effect on the department. Not only does the chief know what is going on, he actually has some clinical sense. It gives the resident a great opportunity to assess his chief and vice versa.

In some areas of the country, a junior staff member is assigned to run the conference. A junior staff member in charge of the morbidity and mortality meeting probably has this function as his major charge. He has the time to coordinate, organize, and improve the conference. However, junior staff are just that—junior. They lack the leeway given to a chief resident and do not engender the respect of a chief of surgery. They are too junior to use the word "experience." They are too senior to buckle under. They are, in effect, too surgically adolescent to effectively lead a morbidity and mortality conference. Only a chief of surgery or a chief of residents is in a position to drive home the implications of a complication to an audience—the chief of surgery by position, the chief of residents by virtue of his case review.

Junior staff members, however, are excellent referees. I have found that they are close enough to the resident experience yet far enough into the attending experience to channel a discussion toward a middle ground. For example, if a resident is verbally cornered by an overbearing attending, the junior staff can "rescue" the

---

*Personal communication from McAllister, Rodney M., Chief of Cleaning Crew, McCormick Place, Chicago, IL, October 24, 1991, as he was sweeping the booth assigned to the Association for Surgical Education during the American College of Surgeons Convention. Also, personal communication from Paul Hebert, M.D., Past President, Association for Surgical Education.

resident by defusing an issue or by raising other issues that may be more germane to the case.

The moderator plays the key role in guiding and stimulating discussions. He is almost as important as the presenter. His demeanor and approach set the tone for the conference. He must recognize when discussions become fruitless or when points are glossed over. The greater the demands by the moderator, both on the presenting resident and the audience, the higher the caliber of the conference.

The moderator must be diplomatic. There are many gray areas in clinical surgery, and it is a natural surgical tendency to feel that "my way is the only way." In the face of a complication in which surgical judgment and practice are questioned, the discussion needs to be steered toward the less personal aspects of practice. A disinterested moderator can devastate the conference. A seasoned and knowledgeable moderator can enhance it.

Whoever the moderator is, he must be demanding, understanding, reasonable, polite, and, above all, fair. He must guide the often heated discussions and must distill the comments into a worthwhile valuable teaching endeavor.

THE ROOM

Morbidity and mortality conference rooms vary from the small to the large and from the crowded to the desolate. The current room I attend has the warmth, personality, and educational aura of Boston Garden. Some of the rooms are expansive. The only other room in which you will feel so special will be at your Bar Mitzvah or wedding. A large impersonal room, however, has advantages to the presenter. People in the back row of a large room cannot see anastomotic leaks and therefore are unable to grill you about the films. Older surgeons, slightly hard of hearing, will not be able to differentiate between ceflaxotixin, cefalaxitoxicin, or cefallaxoticitocin. This too will help your presentation. Acoustics are bad, so you can mumble, and, people being who they are, you will not get asked to clarify your statements.

The room in which the morbidity and mortality meeting is held is also a "room of the mind." When the surgeon enters this room, he should leave behind the baggage he carries during his daily practice. Hospital politics, personal likes and dislikes, competitors, enemies—all of these forces should be checked at the door. The sophisticated morbidity and mortality audience realizes that issues can be vocally and passionately discussed in a meeting without engaging in character assassination or blind devotion to outmoded principles.

In this room of education, it is " . . . nothing personal. It's just business."* When the doors of the meeting close, the educational process begins. When the meeting is over, the doors open and surgical life resumes.

I prefer a small room to the vast caverns in vogue today at large medical centers. Small rooms for the morbidity and mortality conference link us to our surgical past. If I were asked to design such a room (and I know hospital architects at this moment are rushing to the phone) there would be oak-paneled walls with portraits of the surgical greats on either side. Classical music (Wagner) would be softly playing as the audience files in. A picture of Carl Yastrzemski's last at-bat would be prominently displayed. A large mahogany table would occupy its center. Comfortable chairs would surround the table. The chief resident and his minions would be at one end, while the members of the division of surgery would be at the other. View boxes, slide projectors, video-tape projectors and overhead projectors would be built in. Double decaf amaretto capuccino would not be available. The room would set the tone for a serious and educational discussion.

In such a room, films could be seen without having to re-create the Bataan Death March from the back of a great hall. Words could be heard. The speaker, if necessary, could be courteously interrupted. Furthermore, when the verbal jousting begins, preening overachievers could be skewered in close view of their enemies.

Such a small room also makes attendance easier to record. While attendance at morbidity and mortality meetings is not required in all divisions, it is certainly noticed. Patterns of attendance may reflect level of involvement in the division. One interesting pattern is the surgeon consistently absent when his complications are being presented, yet present and quite vocal when they are not.

---

*Vito Corleone to Michael Corleone in "The Godfather," Blockbuster Video, Aisle 6, Classics.

A small room works particularly well for the resident who has fallen asleep. His colleagues can keep him awake if the resident presentation does not.

THE AUDIENCE

There is no more fascinating study of human ego, emotion, and prejudice than intelligently and insightfully studying the audience at a surgical morbidity and mortality meeting. To the astute observer, this forum exposes surgical prejudice, faulty reasoning, illogical thinking, and refined stupidity. Alternatively, it exposes clinical wisdom, technical excellence, and superb judgment. Understanding the audience is essential to understanding the basic dynamic of the meeting. It is of great value to the presenter.

In many prominent surgical centers, attendance at the morbidity and mortality meeting is a requirement for divisional status or membership on a teaching service. Regrettably, this is not the case in other areas of the country. This means that the audience may be small and variable. It will exhibit varying degrees of commitment to the meeting.

Seating is important in understanding the audience because it is a constant. Everyone sits in the same place every week. Why? Surgeons are creatures of habit. It works to the advantage of the presenter, who will learn from which sections difficult questions and comments arise. The following diagram outlines the usual morbidity and mortality seating arrangements.

PRESENTING RESIDENT

RETIRED SURGEONS	FULL-TIME
	SURGEONS SECTOR I
SURGEONS WHO SHOULD RETIRE	SENIOR RESIDENTS
VIABLE SURGEONS	JUNIOR RESIDENTS
PART-TIME SURGEONS	
TWEENERS	FULL-TIME SURGEONS
LUMPENPROLETARIAT	SECTOR II

SUPPORT STAFF

COFFEE

Who attends the surgical morbidity and mortality meeting?

Professors

I will not cloud the purity of this discourse with my complete views on the surgical professoriate. What has happened in academia in America has been recently described in three books.* Their agenda has been discussed elsewhere.† Their goals, positions, and influence on surgical education will be discussed in an upcoming *Gordon's Guide*.

The history of the professoriate is an interesting and storied one. One fact has always stood out in my mind. The earliest goal of the professoriate was to **restrict** knowledge to the professoriate. They felt that the commoners were unworthy of learning. Intellectual protectionism and inbreeding followed. This principle of professorial life was the basis for the inital town-gown rivalry—a rivalry that persists today in every aspect of eduational life. It always seemed illogical to me that the people to whom the public looks for knowledge should have begun their history by restricting that knowledge. To some degree, this philosophy persists in academia today.

My own perception of the medical professoriate formed during my medical school years. That perception was refined during my residency. It was solidified during M and M meetings. It was distilled during my practice. These perceptions are now a sweet nectar (having been formed, refined, and distilled), enriching my professional life. They help me to deal with the professoriate. They guide me. They comfort me.

My own background has also played a role in forming my views. My father probably summed it up best when he said, referring to a friend's son, "He may be a Harvard professor, but he has no *sechel*!" *Sechel* is common sense born of experience. It is practical wisdom—the single most important aspect of surgical care.

An intimate knowledge of the surgical professoriate is essential for any surgical resident. The resident-professor dynamic is critical for a resident's success in his program, and particularly for success at the morbidity and mortality meeting. Professors run the programs. Residents are in the programs. No matter what the role

---

*Sykes, Charles J: Profscam. New York, St. Martin's Press, 1988.
Anderson, Martin: Impostors in the Temple. New York, Simon and Schuster, 1992.
D'Souza, Dinesh: Illiberal Education. New York, Vintage Books, 1992.
†Waltman, Richard E: Adverse Reaction to Academic's Prescription for Success. American Medical News, May 4, 1992, p. 35.

THE FORMAT

of private surgeons in any program, the professors have the last word.

As surgical residents will learn, the academic world is a strange place. It is of interest that the second or third definition of *academic* in most dictionaries is: of no practical importance, merely theoretical. Residents will do well to keep this in mind as they listen to pronouncements, rules, inviolate principles of surgery, and, most important, assessment of other surgeons by the professoriate. These pronouncements are frequently made within the format of the morbidity and mortality meeting.

The presenting resident should understand that the word **professor** came into our language from the Middle English verb "to profess," a term used to describe a person who was **bound by a religious vow**. One can imagine the breadth of thought, the willingness to see other views, and the conviviality implicit in a group to whom this name was applied. As "professors," i.e., those who have "professed," they have taken vows that bind them to a rigid set of principles never to be challenged or otherwise questioned. They will vehemently deny this, yet they know that they view themselves as "keepers of the flame" of surgical purity. They took the vow. They must follow the professorial rules.

The presenter should always remember that, as a general rule, professors have difficulty understanding nuance, innovation, or fresh insight into previously unchallenged surgical rules **unless that nuance, insight challenge, or innovation arises from their own ranks**. Even then, it is only grudgingly acknowledged. The morbidity and mortality presenter will be well served if he keeps this in mind during the case discussion.

The presenting resident should also understand that the goal of the surgical professoriate, to a large degree, is the **perpetuation of surgical myth**. Most of the professors feel that because Charnley Huddleston III said in 1952 that the outer layer of the third anastomosis should be 5-0 silk, it has somehow become an inviolate law of existence. Giants of American surgery create these myths, then retreat to their offices to practice the professorial eye squint, that definite orbicularic spasm that follows any new idea presented to them. One need only to study the development and proliferation of laparoscopic cholecystectomy to understand the essence of the professoriate. Such surgical-professorial action stifles creative, original, exciting, and innovative thought in any resident. Professorial tautology was the underpinning of my own residency. I have spent my career intellectually repairing its devastating effects and assuring that any resident under my aegis understands and combats it. More people have been killed by "Never let the sun rise or set on a small bowel obstruction" than any war in recent history. Surgical myth!

The presenting resident must understand that the professoriate is somewhat illogical. Only under the mantle of surgical academia can a neophyte surgeon review, assess, and indict the activity of an experienced surgeon. He will do this when called upon in the morbidity and mortality format. Because many morbidity and mortality meetings are run by academicians, this is a frequent event. For the resident's own surgical development, it is wise to remember the old Viet Nam veteran's comment about the loquacious grunt who had never seen any action: "He can talk the talk, but he can't walk the walk!"

One final resident warning about the dynamics of the professoriate. Every real professor goes to bed at night praying his boss will die, resign, leave, or be fired! Only through these four mechanisms (the real underpinnings of academic advancement) can an academician progress through a career. Their responses at morbidity and mortality, if analyzed, may often reflect these desires.

Professors constitute part of every audience for the morbidity and mortality conference. They are can be divided into two groups—braniacs and maniacs. The **braniacs** will remind you that the cyclic-AMP levels may be depressed, but they do not realize that the stoma should be proximal to the obstructing lesion. The **maniacs** recognize both principles, but insist it has something to do with their "research interest"* and will divert the discussion to that interest.

For example:
Resident: The patient developed respiratory distress on the third postoperative day.
Braniac Professor: "Did you measure his 2,3 diethyl cyclic esterase preop? (This will be asked as if this were a hematocrit.)
Maniac Professor: We see this frequently in our limb-lengthening patients.

The resident should remain calm during these comments and let the professors have their fun. Never forget that the medical center

---

*This term "research interest" is the hallmark of the maniac. A frequent ploy to evade direct questioning among the professoriate is to respond knowingly to an inextricably difficult problem with the trademark chin-stroke and the plaintive cry, "Yes, that's a research interest of mine!"

is their home and the resident is a guest in it. Listen to the comment, say something soothing such as :

"My that's interesting!" or
"Well, I'll be!" (This works well in the Midwest) or
"Thank you for that comment."

Then, **please** proceed with the presentation.

To some, my assessment of the professoriate may seem harsh. If one conscientiously studies the M and M meeting, I submit that my view is a balanced one. No segment of the surgical team is above criticism at a serious M and M meeting. No title, position, rank, or perceived position should shield anyone from a legitimate question of surgical propriety. At the M and M meeting, the audience should see a set of surgical principles first, and an individual surgeon second.

Professors know that the public will always be in love with them. The public sees Mr. Chips when the term "professor" is used. For that reason, my partner and I always refer to ourselves as "Professor" in front of patients. Not long ago, we both exited examining rooms at the same time. As is our custom, we bowed, as two German sugeons might have done in the late 1800's. During the bow, we addressed each other simultaneously and in a slow respectful greeting said: "Professor." We ended the bow and resumed our work. An elderly couple witnessed this. The woman nudged her husband and said, "See, they're both professors!"

A forthcoming *Gordon's Guide* will explore the surgical professoriate further. It will give the surgical resident a detailed look at its history and structure. For the purpose of M and M activity, the resident must understand the professoriate only in the context of the meeting.

Having mastered the subject of professorial involvement at the morbidity and mortality meeting, it is time to examine another segment of the audience.

The Private Types

The private practice of clinical surgery is the highest calling of humanity. A calling higher than the clergy, private practice is the wellspring of clear and practical surgical thought and action in

America. Private practice has been molded and disciplined by the marketplace. Lest we forget as we extol the virtues of education and learning, the marketplace is the dynamo that runs this entity we call America. If one is above the marketplace, one does not grasp the basics of life in America.

For that reason, it is essential that the presentation lean heavily toward the private surgeon. Clarity, focus, safety and practicality—these are the foundation of private surgical practice. Usually, the private types have no contractual affiliation with the surgical department. For that reason, they can pretty much speak their minds in a conference. They are usually part of any residency training program because they do the bulk of the operations and provide the residents with operative experience. This is as it should be.

Private surgeons are individuals who interpret the rules of clinical surgery along broader lines. They realize the vagaries of human biology and the benefits of dynamic surgical thought. They also believe that no rule of medicine is inviolate. They have developed the ability to adapt. Private practitioners usually do not have a surgical boss. **What a great feeling** it is to have no boss! If you have a boss, you hate him! Everyone hates his boss whether he is the shift supervisor at the John Deere factory in Moline or a professor at a prestigious institution.

Most pure academic surgeons view the private types as a necessary evil for resident caseloads. They will never admit this, but when they place that well-rested head on the pillow at night, this is their second thought. Of course, as reviewed earlier, the surgical academician's first thought is, When will that chief's position open up so I can create my own fiefdom?

The private–professor interplay is perhaps the most fascinating dynamic of the morbidity and mortality conference. Behind the veil of diplomacy and collegiality runs deep-seated prejudices within both groups. One is a modestly intelligent, well-educated group of safe surgeons who have chosen to open their own businesses and weather the storm of practice alone. The other is a modestly intelligent, well-educated group that has decided to assume the mantle of the professoriate as a vehicle for practice. The reality for both is somewhere in between.

In the conference, the private surgeons think that volvulus is a Roman god and that DNA is an organization. They find it impossible to differentiate Melmac, from Tic-Tac, from Zantac. Nevertheless, the private types are a vital link to surgical reality in an academic medical center.

Tweeners

Unfortunately, tweeners represent the smallest group at the morbidity and mortality audience. They are professors with a clinical feel or private clinicians with an academic view. Tweeners are the closest thing to real surgeons in any medical center. They are current, concerned, interested, and, above all, have the ability to review their own complications without prejudice.

They represent the surgical middle ground that all smart surgeons recognize as the rudder guiding the surgical ship. This group of surgeons has a current and balanced view of the discipline. They recognize myth and gimmick. They do not cave in to whim or impulse nor are they frozen by academic feat.

I met a tweener once.

The Surgical Lumpenproletariat

The lumpenproletariat are the surgically disenfranchised who make up a large portion of many morbidity and mortality conferences. This group includes:

1. Surgeons seeking continuing medical education credits.
Medical centers continue to perpetuate the myth of the value of continuing medical education. Of all the hours in the surgical week, the only hour for which such credit should be offered is the surgical morbidity and mortality meeting. It remains the only meeting where error of thought is reviewed and discussed. That is the essence of true education.

2. Surgeons new to the staff getting the "lay of the land"
New faces constantly appear at most medical centers, usually in July. Newly appointed surgeons find it valuable to demonstrate their newly acquired knowledge to newly appointed residents. The meeting gives them a forum.

3. Discredited surgeons groping for respectability
Let's face it—not all surgeons are Nobel material. If a surgeon has had problems, the meeting gives him a forum for demonstrating

that if he cannot diagnose appendicitis, at least he can tell someone else how to!

4. Retired surgeons keeping up appearances

The meeting is a haven for surgical retirees, mainly for social reasons.

5. Nonproductive academicians who must be there

Despite the medical economics of the day, it is an inviolate rule of surgical academia that surgical departments generate positions exponentially. New professors appoint fellows who appoint research associates who appoint liaison nurses who appoint nurse practitioners who appoint physicians' assistants who appoint..... you get the idea. These academic *nachschleppers* are part of every division. They attend the meeting for various reasons. Some attend to "keep their hand" in clinical medicine. Others attend to justify their existence in the division and project an aura of involvement.

6. Nurses, students, guests, and support staff

Many people are involved in a surgical service. It is appropriate that these people be at the meeting. It is inappropriate, however, for them to comment unless specifically called upon to do so. One bares his surgical soul to colleagues who have been there, not to limited participants who may see only one facet of a difficult situation.

From the perspective of the resident-presenter, the lumpenproletariat are the counterparts of extras in a movie. They fill in the background against which the drama of the conference unfolds. If central casting were to call for a group of medical looking types, this is the crew they would produce.

The oak-paneled room is ready. The audience is seated. The moderator has made his announcements. The stage is set.

Is the resident prepared to present at the surgical morbidity and mortality conference? Let us examine the key elements of a successful surgical morbidity and mortality conference presentation.

4

The Case Presentation

The key to a successful morbidity and mortality meeting is perfect case preparation by the presenting resident. If the purpose of the morbidity and mortality meeting is to refine surgical thought, the catalyst for that refinement is a well-presented case. There are several requirements for a well-presented case.

PREPARATION

Any resident presenting a case who does not thoroughly and comprehensively know the case, including the main issues and controversies surrounding the complication to be presented, should not be presenting the case.

The most senior resident involved in the care of the patient should present the case. If that happens to be an intern, then he should present. No resident should be denied the experience of presenting a case because of his position.

The resident should conduct himself as if he were the attending surgeon, responsible for every facet of the case. If a resident acts like this in a conference, maybe he will be able to act like this in the real world of clinical surgery where, in fact, he is responsible.

One cannot prepare for a case 5 minutes before the meeting. Spare me the litany of sleepless nights, unreasonable call schedules, and familial obligations! A team takes a human to the operating room and now brown fluid is coming out of an area not used to brown fluid. The resident is obligated, as the presenter, to prepare a factual, concise, and lucid précis of the events leading up to the appearance of brown fluid and how it was managed. Preparation takes time. The coordination, assimilation and review of data take time. How is this done? The first step is attentive data retrieval.

DATA RETRIEVAL

We practice surgery in a mobile world. People travel, move, relocate, and become displaced. Because of that, they wind up in our hospitals, having had an illness or surgery in another city, state, or country. If a complication develops, the nature of those illnesses becomes a key part of the presentation. Obtaining this data is a challenging but by no means an insurmountable task. It requires a knowledge of the discipline of emporiatrics,* and the will to obtain reliable information.

To effectively present the case, all of the facts must be assembled. There is a prejudice among house staff, perpetrated by narrow-minded attendings, that because a patient had a previous operation, the data are lost or irretrievable. Such data are essential to a case presentation. At the morbidity and mortality meeting, the usual responses to a query about missing data are:

1. That was five years ago.
2. That was in Ohio.
3. The pathology was unavailable.
4. We do not know the nature of that operation.

Once a resident or staff member hurls these excuses at the audience, the entire presentation becomes suspect. These statements mean that the presenting parties have no real interest in assembling

---

*Emporiatrics is the study of diseases of a traveling population. The discipline requires a global view of disease, as well as a global view of data retrieval.

the case in a presentable manner. Are they ignorant or just lazy? They are probably ignorant of the four "Fs" of surgical historical data retrieval.

The Four Fs

1. Fone. Here we are in the 1990s, able to place two men into orbit to fix a satellite. Why, then, cannot a resident pick up a telephone (charging the cost of the call to the department) and call a record room in another city for operative facts?

Why, then, cannot an interested resident call a surgeon in another city and say, "Dr. Smith, we have Paul Costner here in the ER, could you tell us what was done a few years ago?'

The telephone is a great ally in retrieval of data for patients who cannot give a history, whose history is suspect, whose previous surgeries are not remembered, or whose previous surgeries are suspect.

2. FAX. Not only can we get medical records types to read to us over the phone, but we can actually obtain these documents by the Fax machine. Operative reports, clinic visits, pathology reports, or x-ray reports can all be faxed to the appropriate place. A Fax machine is an essential tool in medical practice today. (I can hear the groans!) Every housestaff lounge, surgeons' lounge, department headquarters, or resident office should have one for this purpose. Even the dreaded "release of record" form can be faxed to the record rooms around the world. There is not a medical records person alive who can stone-wall the directive, "Look this is a medical emergency. Please fax that operative report now or I'll have to page your supervisor." This works every time, even though it is not really an emergency and the responsible resident just wants to look good at the conference.

People are amazed that the appendectomy was never done, that there was some real question as to whether or not Crohn's disease was present, or that there were no findings of a bowel obstruction at the surgery for a bowel obstruction. These are significant points, all of which are retrievable with enthusiasm and tenacity on the part of the resident.

3. **Fellowship.** This word was in vogue in the halcyon (not halcion) days of American surgery. There was a time when the discipline of surgery was a calling rather than a trade. Fellowship was a feeling of camaraderie among surgeons that led to *esprit de corps*, a sense of mutual respect, and, most important, a sense of brotherly (or sisterly) helpfulness. If one were to call a surgeon in another city, that spirit of fellowship would mean that the doctor would take the time to recollect the case, share the problems encountered in performing or diagnosing the problem, and would then help the caller shed new light on the complication with which he was wrestling.

Today, however, in the hypermetabolic litigation cyclone swirling about each and every complication, or "maloccurrence" as the semanticists say, such calls may be regarded as nuisance calls unworthy of a response.

Most knowledgeable surgeons, however, usually respond to such calls. If cooperative, they can shed light on a complication, because many of the facts or thoughts may not be evident in the records.

Using the fellowship of surgery, even though it is a somewhat outmoded and dying element of our practices, can be very helpful in assessing a complication arising from a procedure performed elsewhere.

4. **Fed Ex.** Was it cancer? Was it Crohn's? The presenting resident would be prudent to call and get the slides from the pathology department of the original facility. Call and get the entire record if there is too much to fax. How about x-rays? They can be shipped overnight. Why the "Collected Hits of Richard Clayderman" arrives next-day air, and yet the critical CT scan of a moribund patient languishes in a basement gathering dust is the kind of surgical dilemma the professoriate should be working on! The resident's department should absorb these expenses, since such activity is essential to the most important educational undertaking of the surgical week.

These four Fs are not new pronouncements in surgical education. They are basic tools for concerned residents to assemble the facts of a case. I am amazed at the reluctance of some residents or attendings to get records and slides. They accept as cant anything that was stated or said. It is similar to the constant reference to "landmark papers" in the literature, some of which, if retrieved and read, really do not make much sense.

THE CASE PRESENTATION

The most astonishing data retrieval episode in the history of morbidity and mortality conferences involved a young woman who was told that she had had an appendectomy, yet "nothing had been removed." This took place in Telingha, a city in the Tsinghaii province in northern China. She was in a Boston hospital emergency room with right lower quadrant pain in the pre-fax days. As the workup evolved, a particularly keen resident contacted the State Department, stated that a medical emergency was occurring, and solicited their help in obtaining the operative report and pathology specimen—on a Friday evening. Sunday noon, a State Department escort arrived with a small parcel at the hospital, a mid-level Boston teaching facility. In the box were documents and a jar of formalin containing a piece of tissue. The documents (in Chinese) were sent to a nearby university's language laboratory and the specimen was taken to the pathology department. By the time of the Monday morning morbidity and mortality meeting, the documents had been translated and the specimen had been identified. The patient by that time was recovering from an ileocolectomy for perforated Crohn's disease. The case was discussed as an error in diagnosis, since the team felt she had a perforated appendix or rupture of a previously contained periappendiceal abscess. The Chinese operative note reflected a team confronted with a complex inflammatory mass from which a biopsy was taken. The specimen revealed noncaseating granulomata, as would be seen with Crohn's disease.

Although this data retrieval did not drastically influence the management decision, it rounded out the case, made it interesting, and stood as a testament to persistence and to the value of data retrieval in assessing or putting into perspective a complication. In addition to that, it engendered a "can do" spirit for data retrieval that lent a certain amount of fun to the residency.

After the chart has been reviewed and the data have been retrieved, a coherent presentation must be fashioned. **This should be written as a short summary and should be distributed as part of the conference.** The resident's greatest ally in data preparation and case presentation is a concerned and committed surgical department staff that recognizes the importance of the morbidity and mortality meeting.

Get the secretaries away from the grant applications and under-associate-assistant's itineraries and have them work on something really worthwhile—data retrieval and typed summaries for the audience to help them follow the resident's presentation.

Focus on the main points of the case in the summary.

As our presidential elections have shown, the average audience can concentrate for about 8.75 seconds. Assume the same for the surgical audience. The summary should include a brief history with pertinent physical findings and laboratory data. Appropriate studies should be presented. Even though the presentation may be brief, the presenter must be prepared for the audience to ask if the patient was right handed, had a negative guaiac, or served in the Pacific Theater during World War II. The resident should know this information but does not have to include it in his presentation unless it is pertinent to the complication.

It is helpful, courteous, and advisable to discuss the case with the responsible attending before the morbidity and mortality conference. There are many reasons to do this. The best reason is to eliminate the deadly "factual confrontation clash":

Resident: The tumor was eroding into the stomach.
Attending: Actually, it was transmural but not eroding.
Resident: The case took 3 hours.
Attending: Actually, it took about 1.5 hours.

This back-and-forth correction gambit makes everyone look ill-prepared. Furthermore, it confuses the audience and lessens their interest. Such ongoing corrections destroy the resident's (or attending's) credibility and throw the reliability of the facts of the presentation into doubt. Meeting beforehand sets the tone for the presentation, making the attending your ally instead of your enemy. This meeting also fosters better resident-attending relations, so important in awarding various teaching honors given around the country.

It is courteous to inform the attending that one of his complications is being presented. Meet for a few minutes and review the points to be covered. Perhaps he can give you insight into the case. Perhaps he has references regarding the problem. Anything the presenting resident does not understand about the case can be addressed. Why was this procedure chosen? Which alternatives were discussed intraoperatively? What was the reasoning behind the decision? The attending should help the resident frame his comments, review the studies, and polish the presentation.

What is an attending and just what is he attending to? Did you ever wonder why surgeons are called attending surgeons? The surgeon is attending to surgical problems. His role in the morbidity and mortality conference is crucial. He is ultimately responsible. Request that he be present at the meeting. Defer the case if he cannot attend or schedule it later in the hour. A case presented at morbidity and mortality is a big deal. A surgeon is baring his surgical soul to his colleagues, and the resident owes it to the attending to let him know his case is being discussed. In some divisions, the case simply is not presented unless the responsible attending is present, particularly if an operative death has occurred. A strong conference dictates mandatory attendance by the responsible attending.

The main benefit of being at a major medical center, besides impressing your family, is that a spirit of continuing education and case review is present. Most attendings enjoy this. Nobody likes clinical complications, but all surgeons realize that they tend to do a better job if their work is constantly reviewed. No resident or attending should be reticent to have legitimate complications presented and discussed.

CLASSIFICATION OF COMPLICATIONS

Once the case is ready for presentation, it must be classified. There are four categories of surgical complications:

1. Complications due to the nature of the disease

An 83 y/o male patient presents with a rigid abdomen and sepsis. He has an extensive history of vascular reconstruction. He is taken to surgery where necrosis of the entire small bowel is noted. He expires 36 hours after surgery.

Certain surgical diseases are associated with frequently occurring complications. The death listed above is the result of a complication. It followed an attempt to correct a lethal situation. It failed and the patient died. Even though this complication is expected, it should be classified and reported. Death is one of those events which, if occurring within 30 days of the procedure, should be reported.

2. Complications due to errors in surgical judgment

A 52 y/o female presents with a tender left lower quadrant. Water-soluble contrast enema reveals a free perforation of the sigmoid through a spastic segment. At surgery a perforated sigmoid diverticulitis is found with a large paracolic and pelvic abscess. A primary resection with anastomosis is performed. Eight days later the patient becomes septic from an anastomotic dehiscence.

It is within the category of errors of judgment that most of the controversies lie. These cases give rise to the most spirited discussions. This category relies on accepted surgical practices and standards. To justify in a clear and logical manner a violation of such practice requires specifically delineated circumstances and cogent reasons. Such circumstances are rare. A judgment error is an indictment of the surgeon's thinking. Assessing that thinking is the most instructive part of a morbidity and mortality conference.

3. Complications due to errors in surgical technique

A 62 y/o renal transplant patient suffers a perforated duodenal ulcer. He undergoes surgery 12 hours after the onset of pain. Extensive peritonitis is found. The midline incision is closed with stay sutures of #5 Ethibond and a running suture of #1 Prolene. The patient becomes septic 10 days after surgery. Reexploration reveals a mid-small bowel perforation adherent to a loop of the running midline closure.

Errors in surgical technique cause a reevaluation of the procedure. Reviewing errors in technique are most valuable in reminding the surgeon of the devastating consequences of poor technique.

4. Errors in diagnosis

A 71 y/o male develops a tender right upper quadrant 5 days following coronary artery bypass grafting. Ultrasound shows "sludge." A HIDA scan shows cystic duct obstruction. Surgery revealed a normal gallbladder with no other remarkable findings.

Errors in diagnosis are a special category of surgical complication. Errors in diagnosis indict the thought processes or diagnostic capabilities of the surgeon. Errors of diagnosis involve a much more intellectually oriented set of criteria. How thoughts are formulated to arrive at a diagnosis is the essence of clinical medicine. Because the preoperative diagnosis is the beginning of all therapeutic activ-

THE CASE PRESENTATION

ity in medicine, the steps used to arrive at that diagnosis, when in error, should be critically reviewed.

Some surgeons feel that certain negative laparotomies are not errors in diagnosis. For example, many postsurgical cardiac patients come to exploration when an ischemic intestinal disorder is suspected. If no pathology is found at laparotomy, this, by definition, is an error in diagnosis and should be reported. The same is true for negative laparotomies for trauma. Because the likelihood of the absence of pathology exists, it does not obviate the fact that an error in diagnosis has occurred. You took a critically ill patient to surgery after having assessed him and arrived at the conclusion that a life-threatening **surgical** problem was in the abdomen. There was none. A critical review of the thinking that led up to the decision to operate is essential.

Errors in diagnosis lead to some of the most interesting morbidity and mortality discussions because of the nature of the error. A surgeon assessed the data and came to a conclusion. That conclusion was wrong. Learning why it was wrong is instructive.

Classifying the complication is the responsibility of the presenting resident. The classification usually has been discussed before the conference with the responsible attending. It is tempting to widen the classification of "nature of the disease" to include many surgical complications. This should be the **last** classification to be considered for any complication. The first question to be asked is: Is this an error in judgment or is this an error in technique? It is not unusual for a complication to be reclassified at the end of a discussion.

Before the case discussion begins, the category of complication is stated. For example:

"Our first case is a complication due to an error in judgment—a dehisced colon anastomosis after left colectomy."
"This case is an error in technique—a failed femoral-popliteal bypass graft in a 76-year-old female."

These clearly stated categories set the tone for the presentation and grab the attention of the audience. They call the meeting to order.

PRESENTATION MECHANICS: TEXT, FILM, AND SLIDES

A brief summary of the case, printed and distributed at the beginning of the conference, is probably the single most helpful adjunct to a successful meeting. This is the "data base" of the case and will allow the audience to ask better questions. Rather than spending time on reviewing facts, the time can be spent on exploring other aspects of the case. This summary should be a précis. Several elements contribute to a good case summary:

1. Diagrams
Do you honestly think that an intern knows what a retrocolic isoperistaltic Roux-en-Y choledochojejunostomy is? (For that matter, do you?) The resident should outline gastrointestinal anastomoses, bypasses, diversions, or resections. The presenter can describe the procedure for minutes on end and never be as clear as a line drawing on the board.

2. Audiovisual aids
Each laparoscopic complication should be accompanied by the operative tape. The use of overhead projectors, appropriate pathology specimens, and slides do a great deal to make presentations lively and more interesting. The ability to do this requires a certain level of support and commitment from the front office. Those departments that feel the surgical morbidity and mortality meeting is important enhance the meeting by providing support to the residents. I attended a morbidity and mortality meeting for one year at a university that had its own morbidity and mortality secretary! Her sole function was the preparation of protocols, slides, and bibliographies for the weekly meeting. That was a program that understood the essence of the meeting. It is far better for a department of surgery to spend money on this endeavor than on the room service bill the chief resident ran up at the last ACS convention!

A dedicated morbidity and mortality coordinator often turns out to be the most valuable individual in a resident training program. Such a person allows the resident to spend his time thinking and preparing, rather than running, retrieving, and typing.

3. A summary of the specific operative findings
There is a term used in the production of adult movies that pro-

priety and a respect for my discipline prevent me from using. If I were able to use it, I would use it to describe what the operation is when viewed against the background of other surgical activity. The operation is the central event, though not necessarily the most important. For this reason, the description of that central event must be clear, specific, and anatomically precise.

I am not alone in my perception that a lack of appreciation for anatomic specificity pervades the surgical residents of this country. One need only to listen to a description of operative findings at a morbidity and mortality meeting to note this. Here are a few examples from a recent meeting:

"The lumen of the trachea was smaller than usual."
"He had a huge lymph node behind the right lobe."
"The abscess was massive."
"The lesion was behind the stomach."

Why is it that the pars secundum, fossa duodenalis, and Denonvilliers fascia are meaningless terms to many of today's residents? If anatomic specificity is the intellectual blood that fills the heart of resident operative surgery, that heart is profoundly hypovolemic. By demanding anatomic specificity at the morbidity and mortality meeting—operative findings, reoperative findings, anatomic interpretations of films and scans—a tone will be set for specificity for other areas of clinical activity.

Was it acute appendicitis, acute suppurative appendicitis, acute suppurative retrocecal appendicitis with a retrocolic abscess, or was it perforated tip appendicitis with a pelvic abscess? Presentation of these operative findings should not resemble a Gothic folk tale.*

4. Presentation of the logic behind every preoperative, intraoperative and postoperative decision

Because questions will be posed to the presenting resident, it should be kept in mind that many of those questions can be anticipated and therefore answered in the presentation.

A subtotal colectomy was performed because of multiple carcinomas.
A laparotomy with bile duct exploration was performed because the cystic duct anatomy did not lend itself to transcystic laparoscopic bile duct exploration.

---

*Beowulf, the Niebelungenleid, an internist's case presentation.

The clarity of the presentation eliminates the need for most questions. Avoid terms like "funny," "difficult," "massive," "unusual," "weird," or "never seen anything like it."

Once the case summary has been delivered, the preoperative, intraoperative or postoperative studies are presented.

5. All x-rays relating to a case presented at M and M should be stolen on the spot and sequestered until the conference is over.

"We couldn't find the films" means "We didn't care enough to steal the films."

I am not advocating larceny. What I am advocating is judicious night-time "borrowing" of key films that have a central role in a case presentation.

A pre-meeting review of the pertinent films with the radiologist is **essential** to a well-presented case. A resident will never forget that wisp of contrast material coming from the sigmoid that he missed. Why will he not forget it? Because everybody in the room will leave their seat, view the film, smirk at him, and shake their head. What a great learning experience!

Many are of the opinion that a well-planned surgical morbidity and mortality conference should have a staff radiologist assigned to it. If motivated, this physician can be a key player as the conference unfolds. The studies can be reviewed with expertise. The preoperative differential diagnosis can be widened. The sequence of studies or the appropriateness of studies can be discussed.

> Were the antral folds really thickened?
> Was the fluid collection on the CT really inaccessible to needle aspiration?
> Was the splenic flexure tumor real?

The expanding role of interventional radiologists and the advent of new imaging techniques make the participation of radiologists in today's conferences essential.

6. Prepare the x-rays and review them with the radiologist.
If a radiologist will not attend, or has not been invited to attend, the presenting resident should select the representative x-rays and

THE CASE PRESENTATION

review them with the radiologist so he does not look like the village idiot when the case is presented. The resident should be prepared to point out the significant findings, as well as the insignificant ones. If a duodenal diverticulum is present on a small bowel series revealing a small bowel tumor, the resident should make sure he knows it is there. An overhead projector should be used so the entire audience can see radiologic studies. CT scans and angiograms should be reviewed and should be marked by the radiologist. Who ever argued with a pencil mark on a CT scan?

Laboratory data are another issue. No one can follow a list of numbers. These data should be written on a board or included in the printed summary.

QUESTIONS, ANSWERS, AND DISCUSSION

The dynamic of the surgical morbidity and mortality meeting is the interplay between knowledge and ignorance. Each case is a story that unfolds as the presentation progresses. The knowledge of the presenting resident is exposed through questions, answers, and discussion. The ignorance of the presenting resident is also exposed. Because the meeting is participatory, the ignorance of the audience can also be exposed by inappropriate questions. That is why the meeting is fun.

In a sense, this meeting is theater. For that reason, **surgical morbidity and mortality presentations should be rehearsed.** Just as a presidential debate candidate is prepared for an onslaught of hostile questions of all types, so should the presenter of a case be prepared. This is fun and adds *esprit de corps* to any surgical team. The resident should know that the patient was right-handed. He should know that the patient was allergic to sulfa. He should know every fact about the case. There is no excuse for not knowing!

This "rehearsal" suggestion is frowned upon by many of the professoriate. Some of them feel such actions cheapen the honor inherent in such an academic endeavor. Try it their way for a few weeks, then re-read this section. Rehearsing presentations with the attending or a fellow resident leads the resident to quickly realize that the following are essential:

Anticipation of Probable Questions

It does not take genius to anticipate the usual questions, but it takes genius to frame a logical answer and have it flow with perfect rhetorical cadence. The chief resident or attending responsible should pepper the presenting resident with likely questions before the presentation.

Why was the study done?
What did it add?
Why was a particular procedure done?
Do you know what might have been done as an alternative?
What is the evidence that what you did was correct?

For the inexperienced or junior presenter, anticipating questions is a most helpful tool to overcome stage fright or uneasiness.

Preparation of Answers to Anticipated Questions

Frame the answers in anticipation of the question. Nothing deflates an overbearing attending more than a well-phrased logical answer to what he thinks is a gem of a question asked solely to enhance his position among his peers.

Questions posed to the presenting resident at the meeting generally fall into five categories:

1. Extent of preoperative workup
The resident should be prepared to defend the workup or to criticize the workup if it was inadequate. He should understand why certain tests were done and should be able to discuss what they added to the case. Be honest! If unnecessary or illogical tests were ordered, say so.

2. Timing of surgery
Why was the procedure done *when* it was done? Timing questions usually arise in cases of gastrointestinal bleeding, bowel obstruction, urgent problems associated with inflammatory bowel disease, or obstructive lesions of the colon. Each specific procedure has reason to be done at a particular time depending on the issues of the case.

3. Choice of operation

How can a particular surgical problem be handled in several ways? What is the best way given the age, condition, and surgical anatomy of the patient? The resident should be able to defend the choice of operation with the facts of the case. It is very helpful, if meaningful intraoperative discussions occurred, to mention them in the presentation. For example:

> A subtotal colectomy, rather than a total proctocolectomy, was performed because of the hemodynamic instability of the patient.

> A vagotomy and antrectomy were performed because of the chronicity of the patient's ulcer disease.

4. Diagnosis of the complication

How did the complication present and how was it demonstrated?

5. Care of the complication

The resident should be prepared to discuss the management of the complication and the rationale for that management.

Anticipating these five categories of questions will make answering them in the conference format that much easier.

Fielding Questions

The audience has the right to ask questions, most of which the resident has anticipated. A few remarks are in order:

1. Be polite.

You know, and I know, that the guy who asked that question wouldn't know a mesenteric vein from an esrog. Nevertheless, all responses should be courteous.

2. "I don't know" is an acceptable answer.

Don't use it too often, though. If the resident does not recall a fact pertaining to the case, he should call on the attending to answer.

3. Several questions should not be dignified with an answer.

What type of incision did you use?
Did you drain it?
Did you remove the appendix?

These are the unanswerable arcana of surgical lore. They are usually asked by the least prepared, most confused, easily mystified members of the audience. These were the guys who, in medical school, actually tried to fathom the difference between thrombophlebitis and phlebothrombosis!

When these specific questions are asked, give a knowing glance, use the professorial chin-stroke, and go on to the next questioner.

If the resident has properly prepared the case, most of the questions will have been answered by the presentation. This means that the questions posed by the audience will be aimed at surgical thought processes rather than the facts of the case.

THE CASE IN CONTEXT

Following the presentation, review of the studies, and questions and answers, an attempt is made to put the case in context. Even though there are definite regional differences to surgical practice, all surgeons practice within well-accepted guidelines. Putting the case in context means reviewing the complication against the background of the surgical literature that establishes these guidelines.

Usually in a conference about complications involving surgical errors, debatable points arise. The resident's intraoperative decisions may have been wrong. He must recognize this and walk the line between tenacity and resignation to the fact that he committed an error. The literature may be an ally or an enemy for a surgical choice. It should be presented in a balanced fashion.

As the resident segues to the "case in context" part of the presentation, he should never say, "I reviewed a few papers on this subject..."

We know he has a library card. We know he knows how to use the *Index Medicus* or that he paid the computer person to do a search. The resident should slide fluidly and expertly into the raw science of surgery.

For example:

After drainage of the pelvic abscess, the patient defervesced, resumed a normal diet, and was discharged 7 days after surgery.

Pelvic abscesses are a complication of perforated appendicitis, occurring in 15–25% of cases. Even with perioperative antibiotics and early diagnosis, the rate of pelvic abscess formation has remained significant. It is of interest that the mortality is about 3%, probably reflecting late diagnosis with surgery in a septic patient.

Well-stated, concise. Perfect. If the resident has distributed a handout, the references may be listed on it.

THE SUMMARY

Summarize the case and solicit final questions.

The case has been well-prepared and the presentation has been well-rehearsed. The films have been put up and questions have been anticipated and skillfully answered. The case has been put in the context of the surgical literature.

This is the part of the conference during which the resident can demonstrate what he has learned from the complication. This is also the part during which he must step away from the case and objectively make a statement about the error.

This is the shortest part, since all that has preceded has painted the picture of the complication. Succinctly and economically, the case is seen as an error. For example:

1. Our antibiotic management was wrong, given the nature of the problem.
2. The reconstruction was ill-advised, given the nature of the duodenal anatomy.
3. We were late in recognizing the complication.

These statements require a certain level of surgical maturity, a maturity that is achieved, in part, by repeatedly presenting at a well-run morbidity and mortality conference.

THE ATTENDING SUMMARY

Most surgical morbidity and mortality meetings center around the resident staff. They usually present the cases and discuss them. Often it is forgotten that the patients enter the surgical service under the aegis of an attending. The patient has usually seen the attending preoperatively and understands ultimately who is in charge.

It is customary, and indeed courteous, to allow that attending to speak following the presentation of "his" complication. He is the responsible party. Despite the involvement of residents, the allegiance to surgical education, and the approach of some attendings for residents to "learn from their mistakes," the attending surgeon is the surgeon on whose list the complication appears.

Statements by attendings are usually short, given the structure of the conference. If there is miscommunication or misunderstanding between the presenting resident and the responsible attending, his comments may be longer. This is why the case should be reviewed and discussed prior to the conference. This planning makes all comments more valuable. Rather than spending time clarifying misstated facts of the case, it allows the participants to focus on the surgical judgments involved.

DAMAGE CONTROL

M and M meetings are closed meetings. The term "closed" means that every part of the discussion will become known instantaneously throughout the medical center the minute the meeting is concluded. The tight hospital grapevine assures this. Because of this, an attending or resident will often attempt to soften the impact of a complication. This is damage control. Just as various politicians and public figures try to limit bad press, so do surgeons and residents. I became a student of various techniques of damage control ever since a nurse, observing my central line placement technique, referred to me as "Count Pneumo!"

For those schooled in its nuances, damage control actually begins intraoperatively. When an unusual finding is noted or when a set of circumstances arises that portends a complication, intraoperative discussions begin to lay a foundation for explanation of a postoperative complication. A necrotic left colon may give rise to a subphrenic abscess. A gastrectomy may be followed by gastric atony. Surgeons may discuss these entities intraoperatively **as if the complication had already occured**. If they do occur, the surgeon seems like a genius, and the team views him as a surgical soothsayer. Damage control has begun. The impact of the complication has been lessened by the "vision" of the surgeon.

THE CASE PRESENTATION 39

The area between explanation of surgical action and damage control is gray. None of us wants to appear illogical, ill-prepared, or outdated. For that reason, as we explain ourselves at the M and M meeting, we may become, in a word, defensive. This defensive posture is the damage control mode.

This segment of the discussion is usually woven into the attending's wrapup comments. Despite all semantic efforts to mask it, the attentive M and M attendee will detect the transition. It comes after the science and usually takes four forms:

1. It is recognized and expected, so how bad can it be?
An untoward event contributing to morbidity or mortality is a complication whether it is expected, anticipated, or not. Its appearance does not lessen its impact physiologically; it should not lessen its impact intellectually. Although certain complications may occur with increased likelihood, such complications should be discussed as rigorously and dispassionately as other complications. We strive for surgical perfection. Whether we miss the mark by a foot or a mile, we still miss the mark and should analyze the reasons.

Damage control relies heavily on expected complications from various disease states to overshadow any faulty decision making. A wound infection after ruptured appendicitis does not obviate the need to analyze antibiotic and wound management. A subphrenic abscess after a perforated colon does not lessen the importance of assessing the operative technique. Death after small bowel ischemia does not negate the need to discuss intraoperative decision making.

A flippant approach to expected complications is a key element of damage control.

2. Familial and personal patient considerations exlusive of medicine:
"The family wanted us to do this!" (This is especially true for distal limb revasculariztion.)
"The patient really did not want a colostomy."
"The patient was a super big shot and would not have appreciated a delayed primary closure."
These are flimsiest excuses. There is nothing in the pathology texts that says that family or social position influences human pathology.

3. A reference to the difficulty of the case.
Case difficulty is another underpinning of damage control. Surgery is difficult by nature. **Never rely on difficulty as an excuse for a complication.**

A few descriptive terms frequently used in morbidity and mortality meetings bear definition:

  1. The Difficult Case—a case in which the surgeon's ignorance of anatomy is exposed.
  2. The Fascinating Case—a case performed by a surgeon whose operative load is so pitifully low as to make each case a major life event.
  3. The Unusual Case—a case that exposes the surgeon's ignorance of pathology.
  4. The Tough Case—marketing ploy used by surgeon during postoperative discussions with internist.

4. My experience is that we should do it this way.
Red flags!! Rockets!! Buzzers!! Individual surgical experience is always suspect, particularly when it contradicts standard surgical approaches. Individual experience is a melange of prejudice, myth and fuzzy recollection. Anyone who stands up at a meeting and says: "This is the way I've done it for twenty years, and I have never had a problem." probably has not considered the idea that he may have been doing it wrong for twenty years. His "experience" is a testament to the ability of the fibroblast rather than his surgical skill.

A skillful interweaving of these four elements is the essence of damage control. The uninitiated leave the meeting saying "Yup, the guy didn't want a colostomy, so one should not have been done." A surgeon should do what is indicated, not what is easiest for him or what is more pleasing to the patient.

Chief residents, by virtue of their position, usually weave some damage control into their presentations. They cannot resist it. The truly skillful chiefs do it on a subliminal basis, incorporating specific narrative elements into the original presentation. By the time the details of the complication are presented, the audience is looking at its collective self, breathing a sigh that it was not their case.

Damage control is a recognizable element of morbidity and mortality presentations. It is entirely human to want to preserve a reputation or explain a problem on a basis other than inability or error.

Honest surgeons never engage in damage control.
The rest of us cannot resist its appeal.

THE CASE PRESENTATION 41

The attending's summary is the last word. If the resident has done his job, these last words will reflect the experience and surgical views of the attending.

SPECIAL CIRCUMSTANCES

Protocols are great. Formats are fine. If only human beings would follow them. In every conference, especially the morbidity and mortality conference, special circumstances will arise.

1. Stupid Statements

My mother taught me that there were never any "stupid questions." My mother has never attended a morbidity and mortality meeting.

Stupid statements occur about 1.5 times per morbidity and mortality meeting. The one-half time is the surgeon who realizes his question is stupid **as he is asking it** (we have all had this experience). These surgeons usually realize their error, then say, "Excuse me, that question has already been answered," and then sit down. Some surgeons, however, proceed with the question.

How the resident responds to the stupid question depends on several factors:

A. If the resident does not like the person asking the question, he should allow the questioner to continue. This is known as "digging the hole." The audience will recognize the inanity of the question. The sign for this is the level II M and M Mumble.* The resident should then pause 10 seconds and **proceed as if the question had not been asked!**

B. If the stupid question has been asked by a fellow resident, a friend, or an attending whom the resident holds in high regard, the

---

*Mumbles at M and M are graded I–V as a result of the Tarzana Conference on Surgical Education, April 1978:
Level I—Mumble not noticed, speaker clearly heard
Level II—Mumble noticed by speaker; speaker continues uninterrupted
Level III—Mumble noticed by speaker who pauses less than than 5 seconds, mumble abates, then speaker resumes
Level IV—Mumble noticed by speaker and at least 50% of audience; speaker pauses between 5 and 10 seconds
Level V—Mumble noticed by speaker and entire audience, conference interrupted, leader of conference calls for order

speaker gently reminds him of the facts of the case missed, forgotten, or overlooked by the questioner. For example:

A pulmonary embolus after a Miles resection has been presented.

Question by Sleazeball Attending: How long will you wait now before taking down the colostomy?
Audience: Mumble to level III
Resident (after 10-second pause): Our next case . . .

Question by Nice Attending: How long will you wait now before taking down the colostomy?
Resident: This was a Miles resection for a bulky low-rectal carcinoma. Hopefully this was his last operation.

2. Fights
While typing this word, I feel I have revealed the heart of clinical surgery. We fight disease on the ward and in the operating theater. We also fight surgical ignorance. The ring for fighting surgical ignorance is the morbidity and mortality conference. Discussions and questions about various approaches to surgical problems can sometimes escalate beyond discussion. They can become shouting matches, snide under-the-breath comments and red-faced verbal donnybrooks. Many surgeons feel that their way is the only way, or that a set of beliefs by someone else is patently false. If a discussion evolves about one of these controversial points, the conference can assume a political air.

Ideally, when we attend the morbidity and mortality conference, we leave the cordiality and collegiality of a medical center in the hall. We set aside our natural reluctance to criticize another human being. Our reluctance to judge others disappears. We set aside these rules of conduct for the greater good of the discipline of surgery as well as for our own ongoing education. When the conference is over, we pick up these rules, which we checked at the door.

This is the beauty of the morbidity and mortality conference. It's like those sensitivity groups in the sixties when you spoke the truth for a few moments, but then reverted to the conduct that is non-confrontational and much more conducive to peace among nations.

In many medical centers, a lot of baggage is brought to a morbidity and mortality meeting. In such centers there are alliances of

THE CASE PRESENTATION

power, or marriage, or money. Promises have been made and promises broken. Rather than a cohesive "health-care team," some departments resemble the Holy Roman Empire—a loose alliance of intermittently warring factions. Sometimes the strength of these alliances spill over into the conference, such that two attendings may argue a point just a bit past the level of dispassionate discussion.

For the sake of intrigue, excitement, and fun, if a resident senses a fight brewing during the presentation or discussion, **he should let it escalate!** Nothing is more amusing than seeing two grown men at the peak of their career, red-faced and sweaty, contentious and hyperpneic, shouting at each other about a nonessential decision. It's fun. Thankfully, most of these "fights" play themselves out in several minutes. Then the conference continues.

The truly brilliant chief residents weave a verbal web during the presentation that plays one vocal attending against another.

I have witnessed only one physical fight during a morbidity and mortality meeting. Two attendings had distilled their mutual hatred over a period of 15 years. A point of technique arose during the presentation. Surgeon A spoke. Surgeon B spoke louder. Surgeon A turned red and began shouting about stolen data. Surgeon B turned redder and made an oblique reference to the quality of surgical education at Surgeon A's residency program. Surgeon A headed for Surgeon B. Regrettably, other surgeons intervened and broke it up. I do not remember one thing about Chu Wang's experiments with floating parathyroid glands in the operating theater to see which one had the adenoma, but I'll never forget "The Fight." It's the stuff of surgical legend.

3. Humor

<blockquote>
Misce stultitiam consiliis brevum
Dulce et despire in loco

Mix a little foolishness in your serious plans;
it's lovely to be silly at the right moment
Horace
</blockquote>

Here we touch on a tricky subject. No resident has the privilege of lacing his presentation with witty *bon mots*, humorous German anecdotes, or surgical *double entendres*. Attendings have that right.

As a matter of fact, for the resident, every attending's jokes are funny. The attending, by rank and by tradition, is the most intelligent, witty, urbane, and sophisticated practitioner that ever put on a pair of gloves. This is a surgical law.

Nevertheless, in the question-and-discussion section, humor can be quite valuable to the presenting resident. It is essential that the resident always remember that such humor should never be **at the expense of a surgeon vital to his success.** No one, from the orderly to the chief of surgery, likes to be laughed at.

Humor is a valuable tool to disarm the overblown, the overbearing, or the overheated attending. Examine the following statements:

"That's the best thinking the 18th century can offer . . ."
"Not unless he wants the stoma for life . . ."
"Not unless the patient is a Klingon . . ."
"I tried that . . .once . . ."
"That paper is on microfilm and was unavailable . . ."
"Was that the First World War? . . ."
"Not unless he wants to remain bowlegged."
"If I may quote Osler, 'Intestinal adhesions are the refuge of the diagnostically destitute.'"

These statements are humorous—in the proper context. They gently chide the person involved, relieve tension, and are not embarrassing. Humor can help, but often it can hurt. The resident must be careful with it. Humor should be used as one would use a little known fact about a person—a fact that one keeps in the back pocket to be used only when backed into a corner.

5

The Presentation of Laparoscopic Complications

No change in the recent history of clinical surgery has had more impact or more overwhelming implications than the introduction of laparoscopic techniques. Because many of these techniques have supplanted previous assumptions and prejudices regarding disease and the surgical treatment thereof, complications that arise from these procedures require special attention.

The resident should turn back the clock and relive every great surgical innovation. Imagine being a resident at the Massachusetts General Hospital during the introduction of anesthesia. Imagine being a resident as Semmelweiss was introducing antisepsis in gynecology. Imagine being a resident during the introduction of cardiac surgery. Today's resident is in a similar position. He is learning the art and science of laparoscopic surgery alongside the attending staff and the rest of the world.

Following the introduction of any new technology, there is a fallout of new complications. Witness the complications of the introductions of open surgery, prosthetic grafts, and other new operations. Through a series of complications, the original surgical procedures become refined with the intent of avoiding debilitating complications.

We are in that phase of laparoscopic surgery as of this writing. Ductal injuries, trocar injuries, complications of pneumoperitoneum, abdominal access, as well specific procedure-related complications are appearing at the morbidity and mortality meeting.

For these reasons, the approach to the morbidity and mortality presentation for a laparoscopic complication must be different from the standard approach outlined earlier. We are dealing with a part of general surgery that is only four years old. Furthermore, the M and M audience of today is a transition audience. It is witnessing the introduction of a variety of new procedures. In addition to the standard preparation for the conference outlined in earlier chapters, the following should be used as guidelines for the presentation of laparoscopic presentations.

1. The rationale for the laparoscopic approach must be explained, particularly for the more advanced procedures.
Although laparoscopic cholecystectomy has supplanted open cholecystectomy for the surgical treatment of gallstones, other procedures today are competitive. Bile duct exploration, appendectomy, hernia repair, and colon resection fall into this category. The presenting resident should be able to describe in the presentation the reason for choosing the laparoscopic approach.

Indications and contraindications should be kept in mind. The more advanced procedures are under a great deal of scrutiny as their techniques become refined. Such scrutiny makes it imperative that the decisions for surgery be clearly thought out. The clarity of that thought process should be evident at the meeting. The resident should be able to support the choice of the laparoscopic approach.

2. The specific laparoscopic techniques must be discussed.
Never assume that the entire audience understands laparoscopic hiatal hernia repair or laparoscopic splenectomy. The resident is addressing a transition audience of varying laparoscopic skill and education. Trocar placement, use of retractors, suturing techniques,

THE PRESENTATION OF LAPAROSCOPIC COMPLICATIONS 47

combined approaches—these are all combinations of surgical laparoscopic activity that may play a role in the performance of these cases. They should be explained, presented, and discussed.

3. Ideally, each laparoscopic complication should be accompanied by the operative videotape, if it exists.
Many laparoscopic procedures are becoming routine and are therefore not being taped. Besides, the way tapes are handled and categorized in most operating rooms, one usually winds up viewing the candlelighting ceremony at the Steinberg Bar Mitzvah instead of the colon resection of Mr. Steinberg. Nevertheless, the videotape is a record of the procedure. Unlike the operative report, the operative videotape represents anatomy for all to see. This operative anatomy is not related secondhand by a standard operative report. It is projected so all may view what the operating surgeon viewed. The tape assumes more importance when there is a complication. Was there anything on the field that may have hinted at the complication? A subtle bile discoloration, some cloudy fluid, blood after irrigation, etc. may be noted in retrospect on the video.

Each laparoscopic case now has available its own Zapruder film. It can be analyzed, slowed down, replayed (up and to the left, up and to the left, up and to the left) until some light can be shed on the origin of the complication.

One of the benefits of the laparoscopic revolution has been the projection of individual surgeon's activities onto big screen televisions. It is the surgical loudmouth's worst enemy. It is fun to see the "gifted technical surgeon," whose hobby is browbeating residents, misidentify the right tube for the appendix! The triply-boarded twit who calls you every night at 11:30 doesn't seem quite so intimidating after broadcasting his flailing graspers in front of the M and M audience. It is even more fun to see the young upstart with wet ink on his board certificate smoothly and effortlessly dig out a cicatrized gallbladder. These tapes are eye-openers in every sense. They can instruct in a manner previously unavailable to residents and M and M audiences. Operative anatomy becomes alive, dynamic, and real for the audience.

4. The complication should be discussed in the context of the current laparoscopic literature.
The general surgical laparoscopic literature is, as of this writing, about four years old. It changes weekly. It is exploding. It is chal-

lenging and instructive for today's residents to acquaint themselves with an evolving literature, as opposed to the remainder of the general surgical literature, which is, as of this writing, somewhat static.

Standard General Surgical Literature Titles Appearing Monthly

1. The asymptomatic carotid bruit
2. Morbidity of Whipple—a collective review
3. Ringer's or saline for resuscitation?
4. Operative approaches to hemorrhagic pancreatitis
5. Abdominal sepsis—"new concepts"
6. Does 2-3,diethyl sidnethyl estheresterase prevent carbon bonding in the adrenalectomized ferret?

The Evolving Laparoscopic Surgical Literature

1. Laparoscopic common bile duct exploration—evolving techniques and complications
2. Laparoscopic hernia repair—evolving techniques and complications
3. Solid organ removal (spleen, adrenal, etc.)—evolving techniques and complications
4. Anesthetic effects of laparoscopy—complications
5. Laparoscopic appendectomy—techniques, indications and complications

Several excellent textbooks and journals on laparoscopy have been published within the last two years. These texts and journals are specifically dedicated to laparoscopic research and clinical activities. As expected following the introduction of new technologies, a great portion of the papers concerns laparoscopic complications. This evolving literature represents an excellent resource for the presenting resident.

The current laparoscopic literature is dynamic and stimulating, offering new insights into old surgical problems. The standard surgical literature seems to be recycled surgical arcana laced with "presidential addresses" from various clubs. It is proper that laparoscopic complications and the literature surrounding those complications be approached by the presenting resident with a different attitude. The residents today have just as unique an opportunity as

THE PRESENTATION OF LAPAROSCOPIC COMPLICATIONS   49

the staff surgeons today to be part of these innovative techniques. This revolution should be a springboard for more enthusiastic presentations.

5. The nature of the audience changes when a laparoscopic complication is presented.
Laparoscopic surgery in America arose mainly from the private practitioners of surgery. I need not sing all 46 stanzas of the "Ballad of Eddie Joe Reddick."* If you don't know it, you are missing one of the greatest medical stories ever—how a soft-spoken, frustrated country-western singer set the American surgical establishment on its heels. Because of this, the presenting resident must assess the comments regarding a laparoscopic complication **in light of the position and experience of the person making the comment.**

My thoughts on the surgical professoriate have been outlined earlier in this text. I have discussed how the presenting resident should handle questions from this group, realizing their goals, aspirations, and position. A few comments specific to laparoscopic surgery are in order since laparoscopic surgery represents a special area for the professoriate—an area with which many of them are most uncomfortable.

It is natural that the surgical professoriate be vocal regarding laparoscopic complications. They are the guardians of surgical purity. They are the keepers of the pure flame of surgical excellence. They are the wind beneath my wings. Yet, to a large degree, many of them missed the boat. They regret it.

Not long ago I was at an international laparoscopic meeting with great convention facilities and easy freeway access to major recreational facilities. An honest-to-goodness Ivy League professor happened by our demonstration booth. My esteemed partner and I were demonstrating a new laparoscopic technique. We demonstrated our techniques and showed him our stuff. I asked:

"Are you doing this in Boston?"

"No," was the reply, "We are waiting for the results of randomized double-blind clinical studies conducted in a university setting before offering it to our patients."

---

*Fax 310-659-9603 to request this ballad, also available in gift boxes for surgical department chairmen.

"As Freud said," I rejoined, "Sometimes a hot dog is just a hot dog!"

Rarely do I burst into uncontrollable laughter at the expense of a professor. Rarely do I convulse with mirth and incredulity at the foibles of humanity. Rarely do I experience a Jacksonian seizure in the middle of an exhibit hall. And even more rarely do I lose control of bowel and bladder and assume the position of a spent Moro reflex—but I did at that moment. The answer was so typical and so sad.

Many of these laparoscopic techniques are intuitively better for the patient. Some segments of the professoriate cannot accept the fact that many of these techniques arose from the nonprofessorial ranks of surgery. They have a tendency to demean the laparoscopic approach and discuss it with an undertone hint of scientific adventurism, or worse—surgical profiteering. They veil the single greatest missed professorial opportunity under a mantle of scientific protectionism. That gentleman in Boston is doing his department, his patients and **his residents** a disservice with his attitude, a pervasive professorial attitude often reflected in M and M meetings.*

Ageism, a popular victim-stance in America today, can work in reverse in the **M** and **M** meeting. I would feel badly also if all of the fruits of my career were supplanted by some 35-year-old yutz with a laparoscope. Often, older surgeons, practice decimated by the introduction of laparoscopic techniques, will vocally criticize these procedures even though they do not use them.

The presenting resident should understand these points, accept the rank of age and academic status, be courteous, and then query the audience:

"Anyone in the audience **who actually performs the procedure** got any comments?"

Laparoscopic complications represent a special type of complication at this time in surgery. The preparation for and discussion of such complications require a slightly different approach from that used for complications arising from open procedures. The resident will be well served by keeping the above points in mind when presenting a laparoscopic complication.

---

*I will visit this professor in the Old Surgeon's Home in Brighton to deliver him that paper which will be published in the Inter-Galactic Surgical Journal, May 2012.

6

The Unwritten Rules of M and M

Over the years, several unwritten rules have found their way into the morbidity and mortality meeting.

1. Never criticize the Chief of Surgery.
To do so is usually considered a bad career move. If the Chief says the hematocrit was 36%, the hematocrit was 36%. This is called the "Chief's Lab Data." **The Chief is never wrong.**

2. Never criticize the program director.
This is an even worse career move.

3. A junior resident should never question, correct, or criticize his chief resident in the conference setting.
Ever wonder why you were being sent to the record room so often?

4. Respect your elders.
So what if the guy refers to phenol, alcohol, and phlogiston? He was in the trenches when you were in diapers. Show some respect!

5. Never take the fall for a consultant's errors.
Request that complications engendered by interventionalists be presented by the interventionalist. Why should you have to squirm because Dr. X. speared the liver during a transhepatic cholangiogram causing a 6-unit bleed? Why are you on the hot seat because the rotating resident from Chicago (now en route back to Chicago) placed the endotracheal tube in the right main stem? Do not be the fall guy for another person's errors!

6. Never allow the attending surgeon to present the case from the audience.
Should the resident be unprepared, the responsible attending may wish to present the case from the audience. This bespeaks poor preparation, miscommunication, and a disregard for protocol. The moderator should never let this happen. If it does, the case should be tabled and re-presented.

7. Never allow "marshaling of forces" to justify a surgical decision.
The meeting is for surgeons to review their errors. Nonsurgical consultants have no place in this audience. It is an egregious departure from the spirit of rigorous assessment of surgical results to have such a consultant justify a preoperative or postoperative decision in front of the audience. Occasionally a surgeon will request the attendance of a consultant to "plead his case." The moderator should take control and not allow him to speak.

8. Always discount *EVERYTHING* after the following introductory phrases used by *any* member of the audience:

If you're asked on the boards . . .
When you get into practice . . .
What would an attorney do if . . .
In my experience . . .
In Pittsburgh (Boston, New York, Harvard, Yale, Memorial, etc.) we . . .
When I was a resident . . .

7

Dress and Demeanor

My own views on dress for residents stem from my own development in the 60s. Those years were the transition years between interns looking like Dr. Kildare and interns looking like Dr. Dre. During those years, hair became longer and dress became a bit more creative. Bell-bottoms were probably the first departure from standard hospital whites. The Armani concept of tie-dyeing was introduced. Open-winged collars and various arrays of facial hair changed the concept of resident dress. Student photo I.D. cards began to look like terrorist wanted posters. Naturally, there were surgical program requirements, but really, how forceful can you be about an open collar when the dean's office has been over-run by crazed political science majors?

Nevertheless, I have always followed a strict personal dress code. As my parents so subtly put it in 1969: "How would you feel if you were lying ill in bed and some hippie-freak-radical-pinko-draft dodger came in to take care of you?" I coupled this with the fact that Halsted used to send his shirts to London to be laundered and gradually developed my own dress code—conservative, stylish, sort of retro-New England Filene's Basement traditional.

Today, there is wide variation in dress requirements from program to program. Surgical residents, to their credit, continue to toe the line and generally present themselves well. To date I have not seen one little teddy bear entwined on a surgical resident's stethoscope. The ponytail (male) and the earring have been sighted, but these are still in the case-report stages.

Whatever the preference or requirement may be, when a resident goes before his division, his dress should be acceptable to the audience. I have no quarrel with the scrub suit, as others do. Ask America how they picture a busy doctor, and most will conjure up a sleep-deprived surgeon in scrubs. The scrub suit is the garment of enlightenment. It is **never** out-of-bounds or inappropriate. Never in the history of the popular television show Rescue 911 has the victim been wheeled into an office and been asked by a doctor in a suit: "Is there any history of rapid change in hat size?" He is assessed and treated by the scrub-suited surgeon.

Demeanor is quite another matter, since it is influenced by personal development, psyche, public speaking abilities, and guilt over surgical ignorance. These vary from resident to resident.

The resident's demeanor at the M and M meeting reflects the tone and style of his approach to surgical education. To a large degree, ill-prepared presentations bespeak ill-prepared ward or operating theater activities. It is unusual to have crisp well-prepared presentations from residents who do not act similarly on the wards or in the operating theater.

The factors that mold the resident's demeanor are complex. Not all of us are relaxed public speakers. And yet, with preparation, anticipation of questions, practice, and experience, one's demeanor becomes more relaxed and assured.

Overall surgical demeanor is molded by the M and M meeting. The meeting is an excellent training ground for board exams, grand round presentations, and family and patient discussions. A confident and relaxed M and M presenting demeanor spills over to other areas of resident life. It is a great asset.

Such confident and assured demeanor develops over the five years of the program, coming to final stage during the chief year. It is as if junior residents are understudies to great actors. Magically, every July, the lead actors disappear and the understudies take over.

8

The Surgical Notebook

No one on my current service has ever heard of a surgical notebook. Before the days of copy machines, modems, and computer services, before the days of prefabricated surgical professorships, and well before the days of grants, there were four parts to a surgical residency—the patient, the ward, the operating theater, and the surgical notebook. These notebooks were given to interns at the beginning of their training. They were blank bound leather books. Each intern was required to draw in these books each of the operations in which he participated. He was instructed to embellish these drawings with comments about the particular case. Artistic talent was not needed. What was needed was a desire to learn and to record. There was something wonderful about going from the operating theater to the notebook, thinking through the case and recording it while fresh in the mind. I would show you mine but it is in the Welcome Museum. At the end of five years, each finishing resident would have a complete notebook of many operations annotated, amended, and embellished by his own growing surgical knowledge. It was better than any text. It was one of the grand traditions of surgical education.

In addition to the operative notebook was a **complications notebook.** In this book was recorded each case complication the intern or resident presented. These also were annotated and contained line drawings, references, and comments. How could one ever forget the nuances of a complication after so carefully recording it?

Because surgical complications occur in set patterns (wound problems, anastomotic problems, bleeding problems, etc.), this notebook served as a reference tool throughout the year. Services often competed to see which could produce the best notebook by the end of the academic year. Such notebooks were also a timesaver, since complications of a similar type occur frequently during the year. The classic work, *Surgical Complications,* by Artz and Hardy began, I am told, with an industrious intern making a surgical complications notebook!

Besides, when a surgeon dies, what will be left—a meager pension plan, a modest home, a few shares of some worthless biotechnical stock? The children will barely remember the haggard shell who kept mumbling something about cases being "bumped"! But the notebook will last forever.

If a resident dedicates himself to a surgical complication notebook, he will leave a permanent testimony to the dispassionate assessment of his professional mistakes. He will leave the truest testament to the kind of person he was. It is his only shot at surgical immortality.

The Morbidity and Mortality File

As mentioned above, certain types of complications occur frequently. For example, look at five complications from a recent meeting:

1. Pelvic abscess following a ruptured appendix
2. Wound infection following needle localized breast biopsy
3. Postoperative failure of a femoral-popliteal bypass (I bet you're shocked!)
4. Trauma death
5. Small bowel obstruction following surgery for a small bowel obstruction

If the surgical team starts a file on each of these topics, that file can be updated on an ongoing basis. It makes retrieval of current, appropriate papers easier. It makes preparation for the meeting easier. It takes the heat off of a weekly deadline.

At the end of one year, all surgical aspects of that particular complication are known to the entire team. Appropriate papers are usually retrieved by the service intern. Division of labor for preparation of the meeting is helpful. The intern gets the papers, the chief resident formulates the case review, the junior residents retrieve the films. If every member of the team is involved in preparation for the meeting, the interest level is higher and the meeting is more valuable.

If the 5.6 million dollar surgical budget can pop for a file cabinet and a few folders, the service ready-reference complication file is up and running in no time! The "M and M" file becomes a valuable ongoing resource for the entire team.

9

Competition

Surgery, by its very nature, is competitive. What greater testimony to the competitive spirit than going into a locker room, putting on a uniform, referring to the basic unit as a team, and even referring to the object of that team as "the players"? It is us against them, the "them" being the vagaries of surgical pathology. We like to win! Competition is an important part of the spirit of the morbidity and mortality meeting. It can be used as a valuable teaching tool by engendering a healthy competitive spirit among the various surgical teams.

Most surgical services are divided into teams often from different institutions. This is true in the larger East Coast metropolitan areas. Usually a combined morbidity and mortality meeting is held. The natural pride of being associated with a service, school, or institution stimulates competition within the conference setting. The uninitiated may wonder how competition enters into what is basically an educational meeting. The essence of morbidity and mortality competition is that one team outshines the other by better presentations, better preparation, and a more polished approach to the meeting.

The "pyramid system" of resident promotions was the flash point of morbidity and mortality competition. Evidently the research psychologists, educational professors, and resident protectionists felt that this was a "stressful" way to conduct surgical education. It has fallen by the wayside. Say what you will about that system, it refined competition on the surgical service to a very basic goal—job security. The more a resident outshone his peers, the more job security he had. The morbidity and mortality meeting was often the defining moment for residents anxious to keep their jobs. They had to shine at that meeting. If they did not, someone else surely would.

Although this vehicle for morbidity and mortality competition no longer exists, it still can be used as a stimulus for better presentations. I envision a morbidity and mortality meeting in which surgical teams compete against each other in the above fashion, culminating in an end-of-the-year award for the best morbidity and mortality presentations. This reflects that work of the team, guided by the chief resident. It's his year, and it should be his award.

Anyone can analyze a surgical success. It takes talent, understanding, and intelligence to properly analyze a surgical failure. That talent and understanding, demonstrated over a year-long chief residency, should be rewarded.

10

Miscellanea Morbidita

Loose ends, final comments, general observations and friendly advice to the morbidity and mortality presenter, who, to be brilliant at M and M, must know the audience as well as the case.

The various components of the morbidity and mortality meeting audience were reviewed earlier. The information given there allows the discussant to anticipate various questions and comments. If one looks deeper at the audience, an even greater understanding will be gained. Just because people are surgeons does not mean that their personalities are overshadowed by the surgical view. Every surgeon combines himself with his surgery to become a unique surgeon. The personality combines with the surgical view to form, for lack of a better term, a surgical "trademark."

TRADEMARKS

The identification of these "trademarks" is a fascinating aspect of a morbidity and mortality meeting. The event discussed is an error. Each surgeon addresses that error in his own way. Studying the demeanor of surgeons in the meeting will allow the resident to anticipate questions and comments. Of all the areas of the hospital (except the operating theater) where surprises are least appreciated, the morbidity and mortality meeting is high on the list. There will be no surprises if the following "trademarks" are recognized.

Senior Surgeons

The origin of this term is obscure. There is no such designation within any governing body of surgery. No organization has ever defined it. I have never seen such a hospital staff designation. I have always found it quite interesting that the person who first applies this term is usually the surgeon himself during a discussion with a patient.

I suspect that the term originated from surgeons who were approaching retirement. They noticed a decreasing caseload, an avalanche of new surgical methods, and an increasingly competitive environment. To combat the ravages of a senescent practice, they probably began describing themselves with this term as a means of impressing patients. They engaged in surgical hagiography—the rewriting of their own surgical history with the goal of glorification.

To many, the term "senior surgeon" is a term of derision and parody. It is a euphemism for old surgeons, past their prime, who came through in a day when there was credit for past performance. In the embattled calling that is general surgery today, there is no credit for past performance. Getting a current, knowledgeable opinion from a "senior surgeon" is impossible because they are always backward looking instead of forward looking. This is not an indictment of outdated surgical thought, as much as it is a characteristic of advancing age.

Often in the morbidity and mortality meeting a moderator who does not understand the essence of "senior surgeons" will call on them for comments. He does not realize that when these men trained, a haruspex was an integral member of the surgical team. When they speak, get ready for a mish-mash of myth, outdated practice, folklore, and the sweet reverie of days gone by. If there were boards in nostalgia, these guys would be the examiners.

These surgeons however, do fill a larger need. Most of them carry themselves well. They **look** like they know something and very much fulfill the television viewers' ideal of the concerned doctor, riding through the snow in Vermont. They are good for the public relations aspects of general surgery. They can be helpful in putting surgical issues into a historical context. In addition, they engender respect for age, an American cultural deficiency. For these reasons, and because they have little else to do early on a Monday morning, their presence at morbidity and mortality is valuable.

Look at the "senior surgeon" in two ways—as a kind, avuncular, harmless retiree, or as a potential science project for your child if he is interested in carbon-dating! It will be divine justice, having recorded the above for posterity if, in the not-too-distant future, I am found doddering around a medical center in plaid bell-bottoms, mumbling something about "M and M." I envision two young surgeons looking at me quizzically and saying, "What can happen to a person!"

Screamers

There was a kid in the fourth grade at the John Greenleaf Whittier School who knew all the answers, even as the question was being asked. I'm sure you remember him sitting there with his arm uplifted yelling "O-o-o! O-o-o! I know! I know!" Now it's 35 years later and he is an attending surgeon, blurting out comments, screaming diagnoses across the conference room. He is an interrupter, ignorant of the morbidity and mortality format. This guy is not weird or unusual—he's just rude!

If the resident is confronted with a screamer, he should immediately defer to the moderator. Although most attendees at a morbidity and mortality meeting find such people disruptive and annoying, I find screamers amusing. They represent the timeless childishness of the immature mind. Amazingly, they all seem to have large practices!

Scriveners

At every medical meeting, approximately 2% of the audience is furiously taking notes. This is a holdover from years of note-taking in college and medical school. I find it impossible to attend a morbidity and mortality meeting without taking notes. I list the complication, the case review, the pertinent points of the procedure, and the manner in which the complication was handled. This is a holdover from my own surgical notebook. For many people, the act of writing is intimately involved with the act of learning. Do not think that these are ace reporters from wire services, or that these people are writing morbidity and mortality guides. They are learning from your presentations.

Seers

At every meeting, there are two or three surgical seers. These men are the surgical equivalent of Yoda. They are short. They are wizened. They may be wearing golf shirts. They comment on only two issues—cost-containment and ethics. They feel that they have some insight into cost-containment because they bought a house in 1950 for $23,500 and since that time they have felt they were robbed because the bank was charging 4.75% on their loan! They comment on ethics because they see the day in the not-too-distant future when they themselves will be an "83 y/o WM found down whose CT scan showed bilateral subdural hematomata."

Although cost-containment and ethics should not be major themes at a morbidity and mortality meeting, for reasons of respect and courtesy, these surgical seers should be allowed to comment.

Dr. Hubris Schadenfreude

Hubris and *schadenfreude* are two literary themes. Although there is some distance between literature and the conference, this distance is bridged by some individuals. Attending most morbidity and mortality meetings is at least one "bad apple." These people are reminiscent of the evolution of tragic Greek heroes. Those heroes, as they developed, passed through various stages.* There are definite analogies in surgical careers. *Olbos* was the initial stage of happiness and prosperity when the hero seemed blessed. *Koros* described feelings of superiority. *Hubris* followed. **Hubris was the most lethal quality.** It was a dangerous physical and spiritual arrogance that preceded *ate*, the pathetic blind fumbling against destiny, leading to ruin and desolation. *Hubris* was the apex of tragic development. Surgeons who feel they are "above it all" or who feel they are pro-

---

*Paraphrased from Vermeule, Emily: "It's Not a Myth—They're Immortal." In The Red Sox Reader, Dan Riley, 1987, Ventura Arts.

tected from serious complications because of their self-perceived brilliance demonstrate *hubris*.

If one adds the Germanic element of *schadenfreude,* to *hubris,* one can begin to understand the sinister looks and comments from the mean morbidity and mortality attendee. *Schadenfreude* literally means "damage joy" or "injury joy." It is a feeling of joy derived from other's miseries. We all feel relieved when misfortune misses us and strikes someone else. *Schadenfreude* goes beyond that natural feeling to a feeling of happy excitement that someone else is suffering.

Why have I woven a tragic element of Greek heroism and a Germanic word for reveling in other's failures into a text discussing an educational meeting? I have done it to dispel any thoughts of the uniform purity of human intent, even in an educational meeting. For some reason, surgeons have demonstrated consistently over the years these two elements of the darker side of human existence. They seem to converge at the morbidity and mortality meeting when a preening overachiever barely controls his glee as a colleague's elective case inches toward oblivion.

Jealousy, narrow-mindedness, and surgical myopia are the hallmarks of Dr. Hubris Schadenfreude. He should be shunned, avoided, and discounted. By the way, he is known to the surgical residents on the continent as Der Pimpmeister!

Dr. Feelgood

In every audience is the "resident's friend." This surgeon is sort of a "mother-hen" type who constantly and relentlessly praises the residents to the roof no matter how slovenly they appear or how poorly they perform. The residents usually love him. Usually a refugee from the 1960s, or a misguided sort who has recently completed therapy, these praisemeisters speak only to hear themselves. The comments given usually are:

1. "I would like to complement Dr. Jones on the excellence of his presentation."
2. "Boy, that's a difficult case. You should be commended for getting him through."
3. "Dr. Smith did a great job."

I do not begrudge hard-working residents their day in the sun. The morbidity and mortality meeting, however, is an educational endeavor for the assessment of surgical errors, not a smarmy love-fest to resuscitate waning self-esteem.

Torquemada

There is usually one member of the morbidity and mortality audience who truly enjoys the conference, not for its educational value but for the opportunity it provides to torture a student. He is usually the person who was brow-beaten during his own residency. Now he has the ball and the resident has to play it his way.

Fortunately, most of the questions coming from these sociopaths are off base and have nothing to do with anything. The presenting resident must always be on guard for this person. It can give the prepared resident a golden opportunity to deflate, one-up, or verbally emasculate this surgical bottom-feeder.

Even though some of the major surgical programs in this country are based on this psychological torture in the name of education, there is no role for it in the meeting. The moderator must observe the give and take. When a question seems absurd, inflammatory, or ill-advised, the moderator should step in and move the agenda.

Knowledge of these surgical trademarks by the presenting resident will help him perform better at the meeting.

11

The Spirit of M and M: Surgery 101

The morbidity and mortality conference can be a wonderful learning experience for everyone involved. It remains the central learning tool of the residency. It has been described as the "collective wisdom" of the surgical division and sets the tone for the work done within the department. It is most valuable for the resident presenting the case, as it forces him to prepare, to analyze, to defend decisions, and to learn from errors.

I have never been a fan of the "kinder, gentler" morbidity and mortality meeting that seems to have developed as a result of recent research proving that surgical residents are, in fact, human beings. Surgical pathology can be heartless, cruel, devastating, and contentious—the meeting that discusses the effects of that pathology should not shield the resident from those elements. If you think an overbearing attending can make you uncomfortable by being unfair, short-sighted and rough, try a aortoduodenal fistula in a patient in shock at 0300 hours on your anniversary.

The morbidity and mortality meeting should be fun. I hope you remember fun. It is what you had early on in life. Fun seems to be disappearing from medicine today. A rejuvenated spirit behind the morbidity and mortality can do a lot to bring it back.

In surgery, as in life, we learn our greatest lessons from our failures, not our successes. Developing an approach to those failures—how to recognize, assess, and learn from them—is the essence of the surgeon who is constantly refining his skills.

Epilogue

> Every surgeon carries about him a little cemetery, in which from time to time he goes to pray, a cemetery of bitterness and regret, of which he seeks the reason for certain of his failures.
>
> Rene Leriche[*]

Our cemetery of "bitterness and regret" is the weekly surgical morbidity and mortality meeting. Each resident will find his own style of presentation at that meeting. Each will add his own views and concerns as the problems are discussed. There is no more humbling experience in medicine than to have to face a surgical complication that arose from an operation. There is no greater true learning experience than discussing, analyzing, and viewing surgical actions in the cold light of accepted surgical practice. The more rigorous the conference, the greater the purity of the learning. Scorn is often heaped upon those participants at morbidity and mortality who grill, harass, or humiliate the presenter for ignorance of surgical fact or principle. This scorn is truly misdirected. Far more is learned from tough questioning than from gentle prodding or wistful coaching. Surgical pathology itself is humbling, relentless, un-

---

[*]Del Guercio, Louis: After the First Decade: The Raison d'Etre for Complications in Surgery. Complications in Surgery, vol. 11 no. 7 July/August 1992, p. 22.

forgiving and mean. It is not unreasonable that questions about errors should, to some degree, be the same.

The principle is clear. If a resident can prepare the case, answer the questions, defend the action, assess the error, and overcome the barbed question, he will have learned a great life lesson.

Learning this lesson will make him much more than a better surgeon,

It will make him a better person.

Appendix 1: Richard Yee

July 1, 1973 was a stifling hot and humid Boston morning. I had been an intern exactly 47 minutes when a disheveled and foul-smelling senior resident looked at me and said, "Gordon, go to O.R. #4 and do an appendectomy."

Standing there in crisply starched white pants and coat with four uniforms slung over my shoulder, I said "But, I never . . ."

"Just go down there and do it. Rankin will take you through it."

Forty minutes later, I found O.R. #4. Those of you who have never been in a Boston teaching hospital are probably not familiar with the architectural concept of "building on." "Building on" over 175 years leads to the following unique architectural details:

1. Blind corridors
2. Floors that change number without warning
3. Corridors that lead to boiler rooms

4. Stacked pipes that are color coded
5. Color-coded linoleum floor stripes
6. Patients wandering aimlessly with "return to Psych-B" emblazoned on a bathrobe six sizes too small
7. Workers wandering aimlessly
8. Pools of strange liquid on the floor
9. Ancient pressure gauges with yellowed tags hanging off of them that read "inspected by J.G., 4/52".
10. Discarded research hardware
11. New surgical interns looking for the OR

I tried my best to negotiate this maze and to find the operating rooms. I found a locker, hung up my uniforms and "Introduction to Your Internship" packet (all of which were stolen during the upcoming events), and headed for O.R. #4. I was told, before any introductions, that "I was late" and that that was not a good way to begin an internship.

On the operating table was Mr. Yee, a waiter from a well-known local Chinese restaurant. The other fellow in the room, Dr. Rankin, had finished his internship some eight hours earlier. He was the person who was going to "take me through" the appendectomy.

The surgical-educational concept of "take me through" requires some explanation. The basis of Boston surgical education, from the professoriate's point of view, is the inculcation of myth by undertrained residents. These residents assume an aura of knowledge and begin to "teach." They have seniority over an intern, and for that reason can tell the intern what to do. They direct operations with which they are unfamiliar and mask that unfamiliarity by the constant declamation and denigration of their underling, i.e., the intern. It is the grand tradition of the professoriate—the license to criticize without the obligation to understand. "Take me through" in the classic university training setup of the mid-1970s means to give instruction without knowledge, to set example without experience, to direct without direction. I was about to be "taken through" an appendectomy.

The anesthesiologist had been an anesthesiologist for about 47 minutes, having completed a year of internal medicine the prior evening. He had a book propped up at the head of the table and was frantically assembling small vials of drugs. The book was *Introduction to Anesthesia* by Dripps, Eckenhoff and Vandam.

Mr. Yee appeared to be asleep. The case itself was human physiology gone awry. The only thing more awry was the knowledge of the operating team. There was bleeding, shouting, identification of structures, misidentification of structures, sweating, hollering, more bleeding, and some laughing. There was the identification of pus, stool, tenia, cecum, and some swollen tubular structure that was eventually removed. Calling this event an operation is akin to calling a Claymore mine explosion "directed force blast entropy." Of course, the patient was moving during the entire case. The muscles were rigid. The field was in motion. The "team" was bewildered. No one in the room had any idea of what he was doing. True to the Boston surgical tradition, no one said "stop, we need help."

Having been "taken through" this ordeal, the final comment by Dr. Rankin was, "This guy's headed for M and M. Gordon, you better get ready." As I look back on my own surgical career, this statement became the seminal force driving my own surgical education.

Mr. Yee subsequently developed a pelvic abscess, a small bowel obstruction, a cecal fistula, a wound infection, and a brachial nerve palsy. He left the hospital 11 weeks and two operations after the original procedure. He was wearing a colostomy bag over his cecal fistula at the time of discharge.

Shortly after he developed his first complication—a pelvic abscess—the chief resident told me to present the case at the "M and M" meeting. My first question was, "What is an M and M?" I asked what it involved. He told me merely to "discuss the case." Having great faith in human nature (and, at that time, having no insight into the machinations of the Boston surgical mind), I proceeded, the following Monday morning, to do just that.

In a leisurely, story-type manner at 0730 hours on a Monday morning in late July 1973, I delivered my first morbidity and mortality presentation.

The morbidity and mortality meeting in Boston teaching hospitals, in those days, was a combination of the Nazi court system, the Inquisition, and the McCarthy hearings. I am sure the storied history of New England witchcraft persecution was the founding principle of the meeting. In the front row were various distinguished rhinophymic men, all wearing 40-pound wing-tip shoes and corduroy coats (even in July) with patches on the elbows. None of them looked like my uncle Sid.

They had me for breakfast that morning.

I knew nothing. I knew few of the important details of the case, of the operation, or of the approach to any of the problems that the patient experienced. It was the most humiliating and demeaning experience of my life. Frankly, I was angry, not so much for having had my ignorance exposed, but because the attending, resident, and staff hierarchy never told me that the morbidity and mortality meeting had a definite format that required preparation.

I came to realize that the template for presenting successfully at the meeting was the same template for the acquisition of all surgical knowledge during a residency. That template consisted of preparation, anticipation, and library research. Preparing for surgery and clinical work became intimately related to preparing for this weekly meeting.

My ignorance and humiliation were cathartic. Ancient heroes went through a process to become true heroes. A key element to that process was acquiring hubris—a dangerous physical, intellectual, and spiritual arrogance borne of a sense of supreme knowledge or ability. Hubris was a character flaw leading to ruin. The morbidity and mortality meeting rids the resident and the surgeon of hubris. This dynamic works.

Every time I pass that Chinese restaurant on the way to visit my home town, I think of Richard Yee, his ruptured appendix, and that morbidity and mortality meeting. I think of the events that led me to view that meeting and that hour as an essential element of surgical education. Although I was done a great disservice by the surgical hierarchy, I took it upon myself, since that time, to plan for each and every meeting. That meeting, over twenty years ago, I am sure, planted the seed for this guide.

Appendix 2:
The M and M Checklist

1. Data retrieved
2. Summary prepared and typed; audiovisuals prepared.
3. Films retrieved, reviewed with radiologist, then locked up
4. Attending surgeon notified that complication is to be presented
5. List of potential questions drawn up and discussed with attending
6. Category of complication decided
7. Radiologist and pathologist notified that case is to be presented
8. Literature reviewed; case put in context of surgical literature
9. Packet of pertinent papers filed in service complications notebook
10. Shirt retrieved from cleaner

Appendix 3: How to Make M and M More Interesting: A 10-Point Plan

1. An inexpensive desktop computer, a responsible intern, and the pearls from the meeting lead to an informative newsweekly for the department of surgery.
Here is the first headline:

> Cecal Closure to Dr. Feldman: Drain Me!

2. Wide distribution and use of Gordon's Guide will lead to a reexamination of the M and M meeting in every surgical program throughout the world.

The distilled wisdom, the prescient comments, the crystalline insights in this text will enhance surgical education for the ages. The calibre of the presentations will escalate. Residents will realize that the focus of the meeting will be their presentations. A spirit of competition will develop. It will look great on the C.V.—Recipient, Gordon Award, 1998.

3. Attendance at the M and M meeting should be a divisional requirement for those surgeons on a teaching service.
Since medicine today has so many requirements, this onerous idea can be circumvented by linking staff re-appointment to the meeting. Why should staff re-appointment be linked to attendance at the Emeritus Parking Committee meetings and not to M and M?

4. Hire an M and M secretary
The sole responsibility is this meeting (prepare protocols, get audiovisual aids, etc.). Take the money for "The effects of 2,3, diethyl 4 methyl 6 mercaptopurine on the reperfused Wistar rat utricle" study and hire this person!

5. Rotate the moderator
This should be done at least four times a year. It is interesting and informative to see how members of the division handle the task. It stimulates interest in the audience.

6. Collect several complications of the same type and present a "mini-conference"
Not long ago, by accident, three complications of mesenteric ischemia were presented. The presentations were fragmented, but could easily have been synthesized into an interesting mini-conference on this difficult surgical problem. Since common complications occur frequently, this is easy to do.

7. During a slow week (few complications), schedule a debate on a controversial surgical topic related to complications
For example, "The second-look procedure is an outdated concept" or "Needle catheter drainage is superior to reoperation for mesenteric abscesses."

8. Play the game "board busters"
Ten board questions arising out of every M and M meeting are placed on file cards, distributed and drawn randomly throughout the year.

9. Hold a reversal day

The attendings present the complications and the residents act as the attendings. This has potential. Let's see if that guy really can trace the fascial attachments of the pineal!

10. Host a "brown helmet" award dinner

The "brown helmet award" is given each year to the most egregious departure from surgical principle resulting in a horrific complication. This is given to the resident involved with the case who, naturally, caused the complication. The single criterion to be observed is that the patient survives the complication. Speeches are given. Dinner and drinks are served, and yes, it's all charged to the department! As opposed to the Gordon Award, a resident would probably not list this on his C.V.

Appendix 4: Great Moments in the History of the Surgical M and M Meeting

2030 B.C. Hippocrates operates on Epectetus; wound suppurates 5 days later.

2029 B.C. Zion the Elder, Chief of Chirurgery at Thrace General, wonders why Epectetus got ill.

2028 B.C. Hippocrates describes the case to Zion the Younger, who has never heard of such a thing either.

GREAT MOMENTS IN M&M

2027 B.C.   Hippocrates, Zion the Elder and Zion the Younger meet in the Peloponessian Room of the Motel VI in Athens to discuss the case. **This is generally regarded as the first formal M and M meeting**

10 A.D.   Paracelsus clysters Edmund the Unready. A small bowel fistula results.

25 A.D.   The first medical school is founded.

28 A.D.   The Athenian post office refuses to deliver 50 stone slabs, mailed by the medical school soliciting donations.

50 A.D.   The first full-time surgeon is hired.

50 A.D.   (Ten minutes after the above-listed event) The concept of the surgical professoriate is born.

135 A.D.   Galen's mortality for purging approaches 80%.

156 A.D.   Galen reviews purging methods to account for high mortality.

158 A.D.   Galen's mortality drops when he substitutes bismuth for winsbrook leaves.

800 A.D.   Charlemagne is cured of dropsy, gives surgeon sceptre as payment; private practice is born

1000 A.D.   Hammurabi's Code unearthed

1001 A.D.   Personal Injury Law developed

1801   Roentgen is invited to an M and M at the Allgemeine Krankenhouse.

1825   The professoriate invents the idea of the "resident" as a means of pursuing surgical research unencumbered by clinical responsibility.

1868   Koln—the first pimping of a resident occurrs.

GREAT MOMENTS IN M&M

1901   Boston—the weekly M and M meeting begins categorization of complications in Boston teaching hospitals.

1902   Winged-tip shoe sales skyrocket in Suffolk County.

1928   Baltimore—"Would You Drain It" Conference Convenes

1973   New York—Clyde O'Melmehey, tenured Professor of Surgery, admits to an error in judgment.

1994   **Gordon's Guide to the Surgical Morbidity and Mortality Conference is published**

Appendix 5: An Inquiry into the Origin of Surgical Academia

Surgical life at any large medical center leads to involvement with academic surgeons. I have spent most of my adult life studying the strange and mystifying breed *academicus surgicus*. My earlier work has reported on their mating habits and their hierarchical societal advancement traditions.* My classic in-depth study of colle-

---

*Gordon, Leo A: Incestuous Advancement as a Career Ploy. Journal of Academic Archaeology. 126: 123-129, 1984.

Gordon, Leo A, and Billroth, Theodore H. Wahnsinn: The Germanic Influence on Academic Structure. Acta Chirurgica Meshugena 15: 678-689, 1986.

Gordon, Leo A, and Machiavelli, Benevenuto: Character Assassination as an Advancement Technique in Surgical Academia. Proc Royal Society Unemployed Academics 134:989-990, 1987.

gial death as the essence of career advancement is familiar to most readers.* It is coincidental that the end of my sociological work has coincided with my retirement. At this point, having studied the workings of surgical academia, I feel it is appropriate, as a last scholarly move, to explore the origins of this most baffling segment of surgical life.

In late 1987 in Qum (a small town north of Go), a corner of an ancient stone was discovered by a peasant. He sold it to an antiquities dealer, who in turn sold it to the British Museum. Recognizing my own interest in relics of the surgical past, Sir Reginald Treves, museum curator, contacted me in late 1988 and invited me to study the stone. The stone was remarkable. It contained passages in early Amaraic, Old Hebrew, Yiddish, and even had etymological traces of High to Low Middle Upper English. To my joy and astonishment, this fragment unlocked the mystery of the origins of surgical academia.

The stone fragment tells the story of the farmer Academus who helped Castor† and Pollux‡ find their sister, Helen. Helen had been abducted from Sparta by Theseus the Rude. To honor Academus, the elders of Athens decided to protect his olive grove from development. By Athenian law no condominiums could be built there. No subsidized housing for retired Greek soldiers could be erected. No Grecian theme parks could be built. No VII-XI's would ever corrupt its sylvan beauty. This grove was a beautiful tract of forest close to schools and other recreational facilities only one hour from the cultural attractions of a major metropolis.

It was here that Plato, in an effort to avoid rent, chose to hold his initial lectures. Holding lectures in the grove of Academus, Plato became the first "academic." Although we have known this for many years, the manner in which this term "academic" came to be applied to surgeons was never known.

The stone fragment I studied reveals an accident of surgical history that occurred in this grove. It is this accident that gave rise to surgical academia.

---

*Gordon, Leo A: Collegial Death—Promotion in Surgical Academics. Mount Pleasant, Tenured Press, 1988.

†Castor's later escapades are covered in Morrison's Castor, Oil and the Athenian Mining Experience.

‡Pollux is referred to in the poems of Sappho as Pollicis Longus.

THE ORIGIN OF SURGICAL ACADEMIA

The stone tells of two itinerant surgeons, Duplicatus of Crete and Hubris of Phlegmon, who were fleeing Thrace. They were banished from Thrace (by the Thracian Society of Orthopaedic Surgery) for clystering. Clystering was considered unorthodox at that time, since the triple-blind study by Hippus the Elder had not yet been done. Athens, a city of notoriously liberal surgical sentiment, seemed like a good destination. They figured they could set up shop and be back in business in about two months.

As they approached Athens, they looked for a place to camp. Communications being what they were in those days, they had not heard of Plato, his school, or the grove of the farmer Academus. They stumbled onto this grove on Thursday, July 1, 2348 B.C. at about 4 P.M. (This is the date for the beginning of surgical academia.)

As they were airing out their tunics, two brothers, Cimbius and Privatus, approached the grove. They were headed for the Omphalos, a healing shrine on the northern boundary of Athens. Cimbius had chronic abdominal pain. No physician had been able to cure him. Out of frustration, his brother had suggested that they consult the oracle to see if Cimbius could be helped.

As they approached Athens, they recognized the grove of Academus. It was known throughout the region that if you were instructing on the grove, you must be a smart philosopher, Plato's promotional newsletter having been distributed about six months earlier. Everyone knew this except out-of-towners like Duplicatus and Hubris. Cimbius and Privatus camped next to Duplicatus and Hubris and struck up a conversation. The nature of their trip, the history of Cimbius's abdominal pain, and the failure of the local doctors to help him were discussed.

As this discussion continued, Duplicatus made a very significant observation—the seminal observation of surgical academia. He noted that he and his partner were treated with instant respect and awe by these total strangers. This simple accident of time, place, and travel had elevated them to a newly perceived plane of medical expertise. Simply by sitting in the grove of Academus, stature and believability had been conferred upon them. "No-one but a gifted intellect," thought Cimbius, "would ever be allowed to sit in the grove of Academus. What these fellows say must be true!"

Hubris gave Cimbius medical advice. The advice he gave was impractical. It was off-the-wall, unconventional advice rooted in fantasy and myth. (It was tough to root something in myth in those days, since the myths were still evolving.) Sitting in the grove of Academus had given Hubris the liberty to make sweeping pronouncements, to set standards, to decry the good efforts of others, and to judge not from a seat of knowledge but from a seat of false omniscience.

The advice given was regarded by the ill brother as brilliance. How could it be anything else?

Cimbius and Privatus went on their way.* They spread the word that there were two surgeons camped in the grove of Academus. Duplicatus and Hubris became the first academic surgeons. Their fame spread.

Hubris stayed on the grove and people came to seek his counsel. While other surgeons plied their craft in small towns and cities, all patients looked to him for the final word. Hubris went on to found the Hubric School of Surgery, which had four basic tenets:

1. An imbalance of black bile is the controlling element of disease.
2. New ideas are valid only if they arise from the grove of Academus.
3. Work can interfere with your life.
4. Resident education should be the lowest priority of any surgical program.

The proliferation of the Hubric School and the eventual formalization of surgical academia have been discussed elsewhere.[†] My research has completed the puzzle. It has provided the *urstuck* from which all else developed.

The heroic work of Academus led to the creation of a surgical-educational subculture with which we deal every day. Understanding the origin of this subculture in ancient surgical society gives us insight into its function today.

---

*Cimbius went on to consult the oracle at Omphalos. Since he was a case of chronic abdominal pain with negative studies, the oracle was at a loss for specific advice. It remains one of the great tragedies of Athenian history that Cimbius went insane. He ended his life by throwing himself into the infamous Etruscan wolf pit.

†Reston, Philip B: Hubris, Ego and Nestor—Classical Elements in Athenian Academics. New York, Grove Press, 1954.